consultations
in medicine

COMMON COMPLAINTS

A collection of
medical articles from
CONSULTANT magazine

A collection of medical articles from consultant magazine

consultations
in medicine

COMMON COMPLAINTS

Smith Kline & French Laboratories, Philadelphia

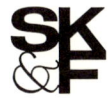

consultations
in medicine

COMMON COMPLAINTS

A Collection of Medical Articles
from CONSULTANT Magazine

All rights reserved.
No part of this book may be
reproduced in any form without
permission of the publisher.

Printed in the
United States of America

Library of Congress Catalog Card **Number 64-17412**

The medical magazine CONSULTANT is
published 10 times a year by
Smith Kline & French Laboratories
for practicing physicians.

Copyright 1964 by Smith Kline & French Laboratories
1500 Spring Garden Street
Philadelphia, Pennsylvania

1,162 Years' Work and Study

Behind every book lies a given amount of work and study — and experience — depending on who wrote the book and how much of himself he invested in it. Behind this book lies a total of 1,162 years of work and study, or rather the distillate of that many years. That's how much time the 40 contributors have spent studying and practicing medicine, gleaning workable patterns of truth from their clinical experience, and crystallizing their ideas about the way complaints of patients ought to be handled.

Because their surest ideas pertain to common complaints — the kind met over and over in everyday practice — we have limited this book to only such complaints. Rare complaints, or rare diseases, are best studied elsewhere, in larger books with more technical data.

Those of you familiar with CONSULTANT will perhaps recognize some of the articles, since all were taken from past issues of that SK&F magazine. We might add that these particular articles interested readers the most among those published in CONSULTANT, and seem to have given the most practical information. Not all "common complaints" are covered, of course, but we hope that you find something truly helpful about the ones that are.

Eugene W. Jackson
For the CONSULTANT Staff

1 | "NUISANCE" COMPLAINTS

S-n-o-r-i-n-g 3
Foul Breath 6
"Low Blood Pressure" and Its Mythical Symptoms 9
Constipation — or So They Say 12
Puzzling Ear Noises 17
Relentless Fatigue
  — Perhaps Psychogenic? 20
  — Perhaps Organic? 23
Trouble Staying on a Diet 27
Disorders in Children That Ought to Be Neglected 30
So-Called Colic in Infants 33
Alleged Growth Problems in Children 37

2 | COMPLAINTS ABOUT THE RESPIRATORY SYSTEM

Many-Faced Asthma 43
Not-So-Simple Allergy 47
Coughs and Coughing 52
Persistent Colds — or Is It an Allergy? 56
Postnasal Drip 58
"Sinus Trouble, Doctor" 60

3 | COMPLAINTS ABOUT THE STOMACH

Obscure Abdominal Pain 67
That So-Called Intractable Ulcer 73

4 | COMPLAINTS ABOUT THE EYES

Vague Complaints About Eyesight 79
Eye Inflammation 83
Failing Vision in the Elderly 87

5 | COMPLAINTS ABOUT THE MIND AND EMOTIONS

Crippling Anxiety 95
Pathological Depression
  — Diagnostic Clues 99
  — Pointers About Treatment 104
Imaginary Ills 108
Disturbances That Call for Psychiatric Referral 111
Bed-Wetting 114

6 | SLIGHT INJURIES

    Cuts That Can Be Treated in Your Office 121

7 | COMPLAINTS ABOUT THE SKIN

    The Plague of Adolescence, Acne 127
    Atopic Dermatitis — or Whatever You Call It 130
    Recurring Canker Sores 133
    Bad Dandruff 136
    Dry Skin 140
    Skin Rashes in the Newborn 143

8 | COMPLAINTS ABOUT THE FEET

    Troublesome Athlete's Foot 151
    Needless Foot Problems in Women 154
    Ingrown Toenail 158

9 | COMPLAINTS PECULIAR TO WOMEN

    Signs That Point to Benign Cervical Erosion 163
    Lumps in the Breast 166
    Dysmenorrhea 169
    Premenstrual Tension 172
    Menopausal Complaints
       — Practical Management 175
       — Hormonal Management 180
    Intractable Infectious Vaginitis 183

10 | DIFFICULT-TO-MANAGE COMPLAINTS

    Hypertension That Requires Treatment 189
    Low-Back Pain 193

    INDEX 198

Allan C. Barnes, M.D., Johns Hopkins University School of Medicine, p. 180

William Bickers, M.D., American University of Beirut, Lebanon, p. 169

Frank L. Bigsby, M.D., Chicago, Illinois, p. 27

Albert N. Brest, M.D., Hahnemann Medical College and Hospital of Philadelphia, p. 9

Benjamin Calesnick, M.D., Hahnemann Medical College and Hospital of Philadelphia, p. 189

D. Ewen Cameron, M.D., McGill University Faculty of Medicine, p. 95

James L. Dennis, M.D., University of California School of Medicine, p. 37

Noah D. Fabricant, M.D., Chicago, Illinois, p. 17

Robert L. Garrard, M.D., Greensboro, North Carolina, p. 111

Dan M. Gordon, M.D., Cornell University Medical College, p. 87

James R. Harris, M.D., University of Pennsylvania School of Medicine, pp. 20, 99

R. Cameron Harrison, M.D., University of Alberta Faculty of Medicine, p. 166

Kenneth H. Hinderer, M.D., University of Pittsburgh School of Medicine, p. 3

Felix Jansey, M.D., Northwestern University Medical School, p. 158

Frances M. Keddie, M.D., University of California School of Medicine, Los Angeles, p. 127

Hans G. Keitel, M.D., Jefferson Medical College of Philadelphia, p. 143

G. Lombard Kelly, M.D., Augusta, Georgia, p. 175

Harvey P. Kopell, M.D., New York University College of Medicine, p. 193

Emory Ladany, M.D., New York University College of Medicine, p. 151

Warren R. Lang, M.D., Jefferson Medical College of Philadelphia, pp. 163, 183

Robert B. Lawson, M.D., University of Miami School of Medicine, p. 30

Milton Mazer, M.D., Martha's Vineyard Guidance Center, Massachusetts, p. 114

Blaine E. McLaughlin, M.D., Woman's Medical College of Pennsylvania, p. 104

James T. Metzger, M.D., Delaware Hospital, Wilmington, Delaware, p. 121

Joseph H. Morton, M.D., New York City, New York, p. 172

Cayetano Muñiz, M.D., Chicago, Illinois, p. 27

Sidney Olansky, M.D., Emory University School of Medicine, p. 130

Marcel Patterson, M.D., University of Texas Medical Branch, Galveston, p. 12

Lyman G. Richards, M.D., Wellesley Hills, Massachusetts, pp. 52, 60

Hyman J. Roberts, M.D., West Palm Beach, Florida, pp. 23, 67

Raymond S. Rosedale, M.D., Canton, Ohio, p. 56

E. William Rosenberg, M.D., University of Tennessee College of Medicine, pp. 133, 136, 140

James L. A. Roth, M.D., Ph.D., University of Pennsylvania Graduate School of Medicine, p. 73

Harold G. Scheie, M.D., University of Pennsylvania School of Medicine, pp. 79, 83

Carlo Scuderi, M.D., University of Illinois College of Medicine, p. 154

Albert P. Seltzer, M.D., University of Pennsylvania Graduate School of Medicine, pp. 6, 58

F. Michael Smith, Jr., M.D., St. Joseph's Hospital, Thibodaux, Louisiana, p. 33

Thomas H. Sternberg, M.D., University of California School of Medicine, Los Angeles, p. 127

Paul P. VanArsdel, Jr., M.D., University of Washington School of Medicine, pp. 43, 47

Charles W. Wahl, M.D., University of California School of Medicine, Los Angeles, p. 108

chapter 1

"NUISANCE" COMPLAINTS

S-N-O-R-I-N-G

Have you ever tried to take a medical history from the patient who "only" wants you to stop his snoring? He cannot give you any information about his affliction because it occurs only when he is sleeping. He has no pain. He will not even be able to tell you when he is cured! The only thing he can tell you is that he is the butt of many sarcastic remarks from his family.

His family will give you conflicting reports of the offending noises he produces — a gentle buzz, a low whistle, a sibilant hiss, a whish, a prolonged snort, or a loud continuing rumble. These varying noises are important to the patient's family but not to you. Ignore the onomatopoeic descriptions of sound and fury — they signify nothing of importance in locating the cause of snoring.

There is no cure-all for snoring. Each case requires a complete history and a thorough examination, as well as an evaluation of the patient's personal habits. If you have the patience to solve the problem, however, you will earn the gratitude of the snorer and of those who are annoyed by his raucous affliction.

Webster's definition of snoring is quite clear: "to breathe during sleep with a rough, hoarse noise, due to vibration of the uvula and the soft palate." Your job is to find out why this vibration exists and to stop it if you can.

Basically, the vibration can be brought about by anything that alters the normal contour of the nasopharyngeal passage, or swells the tissues and thus temporarily blocks part of the passage of free air.

I have divided the most common causes of snoring into three categories — structural difficulties, contributory personal habits, and medical conditions. In examining the snorer, check on all of these, for several of them in combination may be causing the unwanted vibration, either directly, or indirectly by bringing about changes in tissue. Remember that in many instances treatment will fail; but even if it does fail, you may improve the patient's general health by exposing correctable medical and surgical conditions.

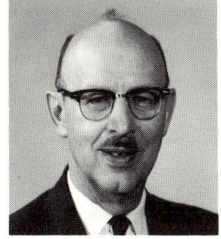

Kenneth H. Hinderer, M.D.
University of Pittsburgh

Doctor Hinderer is Clinical Associate Professor of Otolaryngology at the University of Pittsburgh Medical School. He is also a member of the Senior Staff of three Pittsburgh hospitals — Eye and Ear, St. Francis General, and St. Margaret Memorial. His professional affiliations include the American Academy of Ophthalmology and Otolaryngology, and the American Laryngological, Rhinological and Otological Society.

Structural Difficulties

Mechanical or structural difficulties that may cause snoring are:
 1. *A high arched palate* with malocculsion or facial asymmetry.
 2. *Enlarged tonsils and adenoids* with associated obstruction.
 3. *An elongated edematous uvula,* occasionally associated with a squamous fibroma on the tip of the uvula.
 4. *Collapse of the alae,* shown by long narrow nostrils that flap against the caudal end of the septum on deep inspiration.
 5. *Nasal obstructions and deformities* that interfere with normal breathing and the control of intranasal pressures. These include deviation of the nasal septum or a combined deformity of the septum and nasal pyramid.
 6. *Atrophic rhinitis,* in which one or both nostrils may be open or wider than normal, resulting in a loss of control over the velocity and resistance to air currents and a decrease in intranasal pressures.
 7. *Poorly fitting dentures* that cause relaxation of the facial and pharyngeal muscles.

Contributory Personal Habits

Often, personal habits are largely responsible for snoring. In this area, check the following:
 1. *Smoking.* Examining the pharynx in a heavy smoker reveals a characteristic red, irritated, beefy-looking mucosa — "smoker's throat."
 2. *Eating.* Eating before bedtime of foods to which the patient may be sensitive, or a heavy diet of carbohydrates may cause mucoid postnasal discharge or edema of the nasal mucosa.
 3. *Drinking.* Excessive or constant use of alcoholic beverages contributes to irritation and edema of the pharyngeal tissues.
 4. *Exercise.* Active exercise may stimulate the pituitary-adrenal complex, inducing tension or a state of excitement instead of the relaxation of fatigue.

Medical Conditions

Certain medical conditions may also cause snoring. Look for:
 1. *Endocrine disturbances.* Particularly in the older patient, hypothyroidism and hypometabolism cause flabby tissues and retention of fluids in the nasopharyngeal tissues.
 2. *Allergic rhinitis.* The pale boggy mucosa, with thin watery discharge, may cause vibration of the soft palate. Polyps may also be present.
 3. *Age.* With age come absorption of the subcutaneous fatty tissues, relaxation of the facial muscles, flabbiness of the lips, loss of muscle

tone in the diaphragm and in the thoracic and abdominal walls. All of these changes are conducive to poor respiration and poor oxygenation, and hence to snoring.

What to Do About It?

Naturally, you should first correct any gross nasal or septal deformities. Surgical removal of enlarged tonsils and adenoids — and nasal polyps if they do not respond to treatment — and surgical repair of deformities often eliminate snoring. In rare instances, surgical removal of an extra-long, edematous uvula is of value.

If you find chronic hypertrophy of the turbinates, sinusitis, or allergic rhinitis, you can prescribe mild nose drops and oral antihistamines for relief from mucosal congestion. This may eliminate snoring, but warn the patient that this is a temporary treatment. Treatment of the cause by desensitization to the specific antigen, or local treatment for sinus infection, is necessary to correct the cause of the mucosal congestion.

If you suspect that endocrine problems such as hypothyroidism and hypometabolism are causing flabby tissues and retention of fluid in the neck and throat, treat your patient symptomatically with medications such as multiple vitamins with minerals, the anabolic hormones, or thyroid extract to improve tissue tone. Endocrine problems are particularly prevalent among older patients, but with careful evaluation and proper treatment, you have a good chance of eliminating the snoring.

Treatment may or may not be successful, if you find that the patient suffers from atrophic rhinitis, in which the nose becomes wider and flatter as the tissues atrophy. This structural change slows the free passage of air through the nose. Unfortunately, this condition, with its postnasal discharge, is a common cause of snoring, especially in older patients. The condition is not severe enough for surgery, but medical treatment is not too successful. One treatment that sometimes gives comfort to the patient is the use of "cotton in the nose." Show him how to take a tuft of long-fiber cotton or lamb's wool, or a small square of cleansing tissue flattened to the size of a postage stamp and how to roll it into a ball. Where to place it? In the apex of the vestibule just beneath the dome of the lobular cartilages.

When your examination is negative medically and you cannot trace the cause of snoring to any personal habits, there is not much you can do. You can suggest using several pillows instead of one at night. Newspaper advertisements recommend tying a sling or halter around the head to keep the mouth from falling open. I have not found many snorers willing to resort to such a device, however. It appears that, for these "normal" snorers, the only really effective remedy is a slight poke in the ribs administered by the roommate.

FOUL BREATH

Foul breath is not only the social handicap the ads tell about; it can be a clue to an infection, allergy, or some other disorder unsuspected by the patient and often no place near the mouth. It may, for example, be a clue to a liver disorder, when the odor resembles indol. Or to post-surgical complications, including fecal impaction, peritonitis, acute gastric dilatation, and lung abscess, when the odor resembles boiled cabbage.

Most often, however, the cause of foul breath will be found in the patient's mouth or upper respiratory tract. Decaying teeth and unhealthy gums are common causes. And the teeth, natural or artificial, can be traps for food particles. But there is another food trap commonly overlooked — a cleft tongue. Careful investigation of the back of the patient's tongue will sometimes uncover a transverse pocket containing fermenting food particles. Cleaning out the depressed space will remove the breath odor.

When simple hygienic measures are called for, I remind the patient about the need for carefully brushing the teeth and recommend rinsing the mouth with a solution of a teaspoonful of salt mixed in a glass of water. If the patient is not sensitive to iodine, I suggest adding one or two drops to the solution.

Long-standing mouth-breathing, due to nasal blockage, may cause offensive breath by drying out normal secretion and facilitating entrance into the oral cavity by various microorganisms. Mouth-breathing may result from swollen turbinates, an allergic condition, diseased adenoids, polyps, or some other growth. Odor in such cases can only be stopped by locating and correcting the pathologic condition.

Nasopharyngeal Sources of Foul Breath

In the nasopharynx, a chronic, low-grade pharyngitis leads to alteration of the cells of the lining membrane, with loss of normal ciliary action and a change in the nature of the secretions; unpleasant breath odor results. Infected tonsils may have a similar effect. Even though the

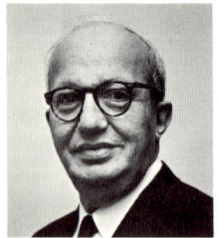

Albert P. Seltzer, M.D.
University of Pennsylvania

Doctor Seltzer is Associate Professor of Otolaryngology at the University of Pennsylvania Graduate School of Medicine; Chief of the Ear, Nose, and Throat Departments at Mercy-Douglass Hospital; and Senior Attending Physician at Albert Einstein Medical Center in Philadelphia. He is a Fellow of the American College of Surgeons.

tonsils may not appear to be enlarged, the crypts may be loaded with microorganisms. The tonsils should be probed or the mucosal lining swabbed to obtain a culture in order to identify the organisms and prescribe proper therapy.

Infection in the nasal cavity can cause foul breath. Any type of rhinitis can be the cause, but especially the atrophic form in which the normal mucosal function is largely destroyed, causing ozena. Cure of ozena usually requires building up the patient's over-all resistance by improved nutrition and proper rest, as well as outdoor exercise. Vitamin A and D supplements are often needed, and sometimes vitamin B_{12} and iron. I have sometimes found that patients can be helped by hydrocortisone or estrogens, though I try these measures only in refractory cases.

The most effective local treatment is nasal irrigation with saline solution once or twice a week, and I often instill Argyrol® 5% solution. I try to limit these measures to office practice, for although patients can learn to inhale saline solution, they too often get both solution and exudate back into the eustachian tube, adding to their troubles. They should be warned against excessive use of Argyrol®. As they do other good medications, they tend to overuse Argyrol®, with harmful results that are well known . . . but not by laymen.

Any intranasal disorder in which there is necrosis or ulcer formation, particularly when there is bleeding with accumulation of blood anywhere along the upper respiratory tract, is apt to cause foul breath due to the breakdown of blood constituents. Postnasal drip, if long continued, is also likely to cause it.

Infected paranasal sinuses can cause breath odor, as can other respiratory tract infections. Chronic bronchitis, bronchiectasis, lung abscess, and gangrene can, too, and so can lung infection by inhaled organisms of Vincent's angina. As with suspected infection of the pharynx, proper therapy of respiratory tract infections naturally depends upon identifying the offending organisms and determining their sensitivity to antibiotics or sulfa drugs.

Determining the Cause

To determine the cause of breath odor, a careful history is the first requisite, followed by a physical examination to rule out liver disease, intestinal and gastric disorders, and possible disorders of the upper respiratory region. Finding decayed teeth does not necessarily mean that referral to a dentist will solve the problem; the patient may also have sinusitis or other upper respiratory infection, or an intestinal disorder.

To determine whether the odor arises in the nose or mouth, have the patient close his lips firmly and exhale forcibly through his nostrils; this breath will come directly from the nasopharynx and nose without passing through the mouth. Then close the nostrils firmly by pinching with thumb and finger, ask the patient to hold his breath a moment and then allow air in the oral cavity to escape *without force.* This will test the odor of the mouth which can be compared with that from the lungs and bronchi by repeating the pinched-nose test, but with forcible exhalation through the mouth.

The patient cannot always be depended on to know when his breath is offensive, since long-standing odors may be unnoticed after he becomes accustomed to them. Also, the olfactory sense varies in acuteness in different individuals. Therefore, you must assume responsibility for telling patients about conditions that should be corrected . . . and for reassuring them when their fears are unwarranted.

QUESTIONS AND ANSWERS

Q. *Do you find that many patients imagine they have bad breath?*

A. Yes, and with the constant bombardment of advertising on the subject, it's surprising that there aren't more breath-odor hypochondriacs. If these patients can't accept reassurance, they should be referred for psychiatric help. Some patients who are obsessed with the belief that they have bad breath may actually create the condition by excessive rinsing and gargling with strong commercial mouthwashes. Overuse of some preparations can damage mucosal tissue and impair the flow of natural secretions.

Q. *Is there anything patients with cleft tongue can do to clean out the food that collects?*

A. They can be taught to create a gag reflex by reaching back into the throat with a finger, while simultaneously coughing vigorously. This will empty the crypt and then they should rinse thoroughly with mild saline solution. Doing this once a day, morning or evening, will keep the area from collecting food particles.

"LOW BLOOD PRESSURE" AND ITS MYTHICAL SYMPTOMS

Not long ago, I received a letter from a general practitioner which said, "After 35 years of practice, I find that the patient with chronic hypotension (90/70) is as difficult to help as the hypertensive patient. Most patients like this are between 30 and 40 years old, have normal blood counts, blood sugar, BMR, and PBI. In fact, every office test is usually normal and even emotional factors seem negligible. These patients try to carry on but are always 'pooped.' What are the causes of this condition? Is there any medication to try?"

This problem puzzles many physicians, and understandably so, because very little can be done about it. There are some organic causes of hypotension, but we should always keep in mind that blood pressure levels have a wide range of normal. Levels around 90/60 or lower are considered as "low blood pressure," but this figure is only an arbitrary one. Lower levels may be quite normal, depending on age, race, sex, and environment. For example, we know that low levels are more common in young people than in old, and in oriental than in occidental persons. In other words, low blood pressures are, in most cases, harmless physiologic variations that warrant no treatment or concern. In fact, they may foretell good health and promise longevity. Recently, physicians have noticed that people with "low blood pressure" often escape arteriosclerotic cardiovascular disease. Recently, too, an insurance society, surveying blood pressures in 4,000,000 applicants followed up for periods of 20 to 25 years, found that people with the lowest blood pressures live longer and stay healthier than those with normal or high blood pressures.

A Complaint, Not a Disease

Evidently, then, persistent low blood pressure (chronic essential hypotension) is not harmful and so cannot be considered a disease. Why is it a recurring complaint? Well, most lay people believe that many vague symptoms, including easy fatigability, lightheadedness, daytime drowsiness, constipation, and postural dizziness, stem from "low blood pres-

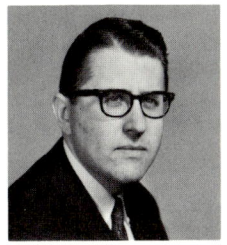

Albert N. Brest, M.D.
Hahnemann Medical College

Doctor Brest is Associate Professor of Medicine and Head of the Section of Vascular Diseases and Renology at the Hahnemann Medical College and Hospital of Philadelphia. He serves on the Medical Advisory Board of the American Heart Association's Council on Circulation, and on the Board of Governors of the Heart Association of Southeastern Pennsylvania. He is a Fellow of the American College of Physicians.

sure." Patients repeat this litany of symptoms as due to low blood pressure so often that it is a real temptation, sometimes, to go along with the idea. However, when tempted in this direction, I find it helpful to remember that all of these symptoms are equally common in hypertensive patients; that treatment with pressor drugs generally fails to produce relief of symptoms in spite of blood pressure elevation; and, finally, that hypotension can be found in very energetic, strong, and obviously healthy people such as athletes, farmers, and laborers. So, there is no correlation between blood pressure levels and the "typical" symptoms of hypotension.

Those patients with chronic essential hypotension who are underweight or physically inactive may benefit by having their general health improved by diet, graduated exercise, and other supportive measures. Others may benefit from rest, because they may be fatigued from real overactivity. However, most have no physical problem at all and the only thing to do for them is look for an emotional cause of the symptoms. Admittedly, this may be difficult to find and even more difficult to do anything practical about. Nevertheless, such an effort, even if futile, is preferable to encouraging the patient's delusion that he has an organic disease.

Organic Causes of Hypotension

Although such cases are comparatively rare, some patients do have an underlying organic cause of hypotension and this possibility should always be considered. Hemorrhage, myocardial infarction, spinal anesthesia and Addisonian crisis may be responsible for acute declines in blood pressure. Secondary types of chronic hypotension include: (1) protracted or wasting disease, including carcinomatosis and malnutrition; (2) various endocrinopathies including Addison's disease and Simmond's disease, and (3) cardiovascular disorders, including aortic stenosis, myocardial insufficiency, and constrictive pericarditis. In most of the latter instances, the hypotensive response is secondary to hypovolemia and/or diminished cardiac output.

Orthostatic Hypotension

A patient is said to have orthostatic hypotension when he shows a marked reduction in blood pressure after a change from the recumbent to the erect position. Some of these patients have genuine symptoms of circulatory inadequacy, usually on first getting out of bed in the morning, and sometimes associated with coughing, straining, or rising suddenly from a stooping or kneeling position.

Orthostatic hypotension occurs in a variety of conditions that impair venous return, cardiac output or peripheral resistance. For example, it may follow prolonged bed rest, especially when associated with febrile illness. The basic problem in these latter cases is decreased venomotor tone caused by flabby muscles, and an associated weakening of orthostatic reflexes.

Other causes of orthostatic hypotension include diseases of the sympathetic nervous system (such as multiple sclerosis, syringomyelia, and peripheral neuropathy) and severe venous insufficiency due to extensive venous varicosities. However, the most common cause of orthostatic hypotension is overdosage with potent antihypertensive agents such as the ganglion-blocking drugs and peripheral sympathoplegics such as guanethidine; this can easily be remedied by reducing drug dosage.

In a very small number of patients, orthostatic hypotension occurs without apparent cause; it is usually associated with the absence of a normal tachycardiac response to appropriate stimuli, and sometimes with other symptoms like impairment of salivation, constipation, or difficult urination. In such patients both arterial and venomotor tonus may be deficient; thus the compensatory vasoconstriction that normally occurs in response to pooling of blood during standing does not take place. This disturbance probably means the patient has diffuse autonomic neuropathy. It is perhaps most common in patients with diabetes mellitus. Sometimes it follows pregnancy or an ill-defined febrile illness, or it may appear spontaneously.

Symptomatic Treatment for Postural Hypotension

Whenever possible, treatment of orthostatic hypotension should be directed at the primary cause. However, there are several ancillary measures that offer symptomatic relief. These include mechanical aids such as elastic stockings and tight abdominal corsets; the latter are especially helpful in patients with weak abdominal muscles. Avoiding motionless standing and heavy meals also reduces the frequency and severity of postural attacks. Increased salt intake (8 to 12 grams daily) with or without salt-retaining steroids such as fluorohydrocortisone (0.1 to 0.3 mg. daily) will increase total blood volume and thereby enhance venous return to the heart. Finally, the administration of sympathomimetic agents such as amphetamine or ephedrine may sometimes be helpful.

* * *

As I said before, however, only a very few patients have correctable organic hypotension. In most cases, both the patient and his physician must accept "low blood pressure" as normal blood pressure.

CONSTIPATION—OR SO THEY SAY

Man's concern with his bowels must be the last tenacious remnant of the bleeding and purging era of therapeutics. Although physiologists discarded autointoxication as a cause of disease many years ago, many patients are still convinced that a daily bowel movement is strictly necessary. Furthermore, they believe that most illnesses, particularly respiratory ones, can be literally driven out through the rectum by a vigorous purge; and that, even when one feels well, a good "cleaning out" at regular intervals keeps one looking "bright eyed and bushytailed." The discovery that a plug of cotton in the rectum can produce the symptoms traditionally attributed to constipation has made no impression on Tall Texans, or short ones for that matter, and I suspect, because our traditions are deep South, that at least a loyal group of Rebels continue to keep the purveyors of laxatives living in luxury.

Is There a Cathartic Tradition?

If you think it far-fetched to refer to this compulsive cartharsis as a tradition, just think back to your own childhood and you will probably recall some experiences like mine. I remember only too vividly that every cold I ever had was accompanied by vigorous diarrhea brought on by a glass of orange juice laced with castor oil. Even now the memory gives me an unpleasant rigor. In those days, visits with neighbor children were sometimes prohibited because these innocents were taking a "round of calomel." If all of this suggests the memories of an octogenarian, I hasten to add that I was born *after* World War I. Actually, even today, patent medicines such as 'Black Draught,' '666,' and 'Baby Percy' are still in use and, although foreign to the city-bred, they still enjoy a brisk trade in certain regions of the United States.

Clearly, these old-fashioned concepts of bowel hygiene are firmly entrenched. They are held with so much fervor that many physicians, and quite understandably so, feel that it just isn't worth trying to correct their patients' habits. Granted, patient preoccupation with the bowels

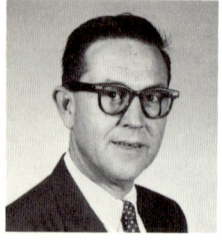

Marcel Patterson, M.D.
University of Texas

Doctor Patterson is Associate Professor of the Department of Internal Medicine at the University of Texas Medical Branch and is Consulting Gastroenterologist at the John Sealy Hospital in Galveston, Texas. He is a Fellow of the American College of Physicians and a member of the American Gastroenterological Association and of the American Federation of Clinical Research.

and laxatives is a nuisance and one that is easier to ignore than cope with; however, it can do a great deal of harm so we really cannot afford to ignore it.

I am convinced that excessive use of laxatives is an important cause of otherwise unexplained gastrointestinal symptoms, and that it leads to much unnecessary and harmful treatment, even including surgery. Many of us forget excessive use of laxatives as a possible cause of gastrointestinal symptoms. What is worse, we even contribute to the problem ourselves — by accepting constipation as an illness in itself; and by casually prescribing unnecessary cathartics.

Consider, for example, how many people are vainly parted from their gallbladders, appendices and assorted other organs to relieve unexplained lower abdominal pains that were really caused by irritable colon due to laxatives. Remember that the "fat, forty and flatulent" syndrome suggests irritable colon disease as well as gallbladder disease. Always ask such a patient about his bowel habits before you order gallbladder tests or permit surgery. Otherwise there will continue to be too many gallbladders studied annually, and too many gallbladderless individuals noisily disgruntled with surgery and surgeons.

How Physicians Encourage Casual Catharsis

First, in a passive way, by complacently accepting the term "constipation." We all know that this term is meaningless as a diagnosis, yet it continues to appear in medical histories. Perhaps we have been conditioned by radio, television, newspaper and magazine advertisements to feel that it tells us something. This conditioning leads to decerebrate therapeutics, that is treatment by reflex: patient complains of constipation; doctor prescribes cathartic. Yet, we all know that constipation is merely a symptom, and that we should know what the patient means by it, and what is causing it, before attempting to relieve it.

I assume, and I hope we all agree, that a complaint of "constipation" deserves special consideration. If the symptom is new, it may be an ominous warning; if chronic, it is probably associated with multiple other complaints that make a careful study mandatory. However, once the complaint is defined, the history of fluid and dietary habits reviewed, the defecation pattern evaluated, and the patient carefully examined to exclude potentially lethal causes of constipation, this symptom needs only the simplest therapy for relief.

For example, a simple explanation of the gastrocolic reflex and how to use it can work wonders. Usually even the most stubborn laxative addict can accept the idea that one does not need to stir up some 30 feet of intestine to move the last few inches. Explaining the physiology of the colon will take more time initially than the writing of a prescription but will save you time in the long run. Besides, there is often a personal reward for curing such a patient of constipation; because of the importance he attaches to bowel function, his gratitude tends to be overwhelming, even approaching adulation. By way of illustration let me tell you about a few of my patients.

An elderly business man had suffered from constipation for years. In spite of (or rather, *because* of) running the gamut of cathartics, he never seemed able to become properly regulated, and alternated between catharsis and constipation. Careful questioning revealed that he habitually went to the office right after breakfast and about 10 a.m., with the slavishness of a martinet, retired to the toilet, urge or no, to attempt to defecate. After a physical examination, including proctoscopy and the usual X-ray studies, excluded any mechanical basis for the *symptom*, I spent some time with him explaining colon physiology, with special emphasis on the gastrocolic reflex. Then I recommended a simple treatment plan. He was to take a large glass of hot water and orange or lemon juice before breakfast and attempt to defecate, not at 10 a.m., but immediately after breakfast. Should he skip a day, he was advised to insert into his rectum, with an ear syringe, three ounces of warm mineral oil at bedtime, and to retain this instillation overnight for expulsion after breakfast the following morning. If nothing happened, he was advised not to panic but to repeat the oil instillation and on the third morning, if there was still no response, to take a 3-pint warm-water enema. With this simple routine, he rarely needed to resort to an enema, and soon achieved normal and spontaneous bowel function.

Another patient, an illustrious local politician, had fussed with his colon all over Texas and the Midwest. In taking his history, I asked in what phase of his life he would have considered his bowels to have functioned normally. He responded: "when I was a cowboy, in my early 20's, riding the range." After a few more questions, he remembered with some astonishment that when he was younger, his bowels never moved more often than every third or fourth day. At this point, I suggested that this was probably normal for him and that an earlier diagnosis, that his "sour stomach" was due to the lack of a daily bowel movement, might be wrong. He agreed to stop his nightly laxative and wait and see what happened. What did happen was gratifying. He found that his bowels did not move every day, but when they did it was without effort and the stool was normal; and his previous abdominal rolling, bloating and flatulence stopped. His "sour stomach" was controlled with a tranquilizer-antispasmodic and an occasional dose of antacid. This patient was almost strictly carnivorous; because of this low-residue diet, it was not surprising that his bowels did not move as often as most people's do.

One young man had dramatic improvement in bowel function after ventilating for almost an hour his hostilities toward employer, wife, and mother-in-law. At first glance, the time spent seems excessive. Actually, it is not, because this patient needed no further treatment. Once he saw the relationship between his constant anger and tension and his bowel function, his symptoms disappeared.

How Physicians Start the Laxative Habit

Sometimes the physician himself inadvertently launches a patient on a career of overusing laxatives. An outstanding example is the common practice of ordering laxatives routinely after delivery. If we stopped to think about it, we would not expect a patient who has been without food during a long labor, and has probably had castor oil and multiple enemas, to have a normal stool the following morning. I can recall throwing a whole nursing service in an uproar when I suggested to my wife that she refuse the laxative offered her at bedtime, and instead ask for hot water and lemon juice before breakfast the next morning.

Sometimes the patient will ask for a laxative she does not need. And, her doctor will usually let her have it with little or no argument, even though a rectal examination would reveal an empty ampulla or only a small amount of feces. All of us know, though we sometimes forget, that there has to be a stool in the rectum and sigmoid or a normal bowel movement cannot occur that day and sometimes not for three or four days.

My experience with the late Dr. Sara Jordon and her treatment for irritable colon convinced me that patients can safely go without a bowel movement for days. Her main principle of treatment was to let the colon rest and to treat it gently. This principle works in treating spastic colon, and is frequently applicable in treating constipation.

Some Local Causes of Constipation

Sometimes "constipation" arises from a chronic anal ulcer. For patients with such an ulcer, a normal, formed stool is painful, so they suppress or ignore the urge and keep the stool liquid with laxatives. This condition is common, and is the usual cause of a history of sharp anal pain on defecation with blood-streaked stools. You can confirm the diagnosis with careful rectal and anoscopic examination and will usually find the ulcer at the base of a sentinel hemorrhoid. Another local cause of constipation is poor perineal tone. This is common in multiparous women who often develop large rectoceles. If a rectocele is present, normal evacuation of the rectum is not possible until the prolapse is surgically corrected.

Constipation as a Neurotic Symptom

It is my impression, though I may be biased, that many patients with chronic gastrointestinal complaints are severely neurotic and that some are even psychotic. Apparently, bowel function has a significance to some that is akin to sexual intercourse. This is a standard joke about the aged, but it is by no means restricted to this group.

I will never forget one fairly young married woman who was referred to me because of "chronic constipation." She avoided sexual intercourse for "religious" reasons but habitually had her husband give her high colonic irrigations for hours while they were nude in the bathroom. Needless to say, this woman was not impressed by my usual lecture on colon physiology and has not yet had a normal bowel movement.

Some patients I have known habitually go through gyrations with an enema tube that can be compared to a Roman orgy. Others inspect stools with the thoroughness of a Dick Tracy and bring me repulsive bits of excreta in bottles, towels or paper napkins to show dolefully or gleefully. Patients like these enjoy or depend on their fecal fixation too much to be parted from it by mere sensible advice. They probably cannot be helped by anything short of formal psychotherapy.

Other patients who cling tenaciously to constipation are depressed persons, children who have discovered its attention-getting possibilities, and the senile and bedridden. However, constipation is most common in tense and sometimes hostile people who cannot relax, who eat hurried and poorly planned meals, and drink little water. Fortunately, this group *does* respond to treatment: i.e., re-education, reassurance, a sensible diet, and occasional sedatives.

Things to Remember

In summary, there are several things all of us can and should do about the patient who claims he is constipated.

- Keep laxative abuse always in mind as a possible cause of unexplained gastrointestinal symptoms.
- Make a real attempt to correct laxative abuse in every patient in whom we find it.
- Remember that constipation is only a *symptom*, so always look for its cause.
- Never begin or encourage the laxative habit by casually recommending cathartics.

PUZZLING EAR NOISES

Ear noise — tinnitus — is a great nuisance to the patient who has it and a great puzzle to the physician who has to treat it. Sometimes it may be heard in only one ear, or in both simultaneously, or first in one ear and later in the other. Some patients say their ear noises sound like the escape of steam, the blowing of a whistle, or the ringing of a high-pitched bell. Others compare the noises to running water or describe them as a roaring, buzzing, or hammering sensation. Occasionally the noise is in the head without reference to the ears, and it may be so loud that even the physician can hear it.

One patient of mine, a young man, complained of a distracting gurgle that seemed to indicate fluid in the middle ear. He was in excellent health, tanned and fit, and had no history of allergy or any sign of upper respiratory infection that could account for the symptom. He had been practicing skin diving, and, as he worked his way to greater depths, the pressure produced this fairly common skin divers' complaint. I inflated the patient's eustachian tube, and doing so relieved his ear noises.

Ear Disorders That Cause Ear Noises

Ear noise may be encountered in any form of ear disease. It takes place in nerve deafness, otosclerosis, Ménière's disease, and obstruction of the eustachian tube, to name a few of the more important ones (Table 1). In cases of otitis media, pulsating noises are frequently produced. And, just as pain signifies irritation of a sensory nerve, ear noise may signify irritation of the cochlear mechanism.

Ear noise often results from the pressure of cerumen against the drum membrane. Water entering the ear canal and causing dried cerumen to swell is a common occurrence, especially during the summertime when swimming is popular. Removing the cerumen with a cerumen spoon or syringing the ear with lukewarm water will bring relief. It may be necessary at times to first soften the cerumen with liquid Albolene®.

A gurgling noise in the ear is caused by fluid in the middle-ear cavity and usually follows infection or allergy in the nose, sinuses, throat, or

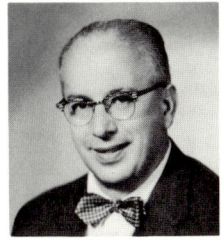

Noah D. Fabricant, M.D.
Chicago, Illinois

Doctor Fabricant is editor in charge of otolaryngology of the EYE, EAR, NOSE AND THROAT MONTHLY and a contributing editor to the AMERICAN JOURNAL OF MEDICAL SCIENCES. He is a member of the American Academy of Ophthalmology and Otolaryngology. He was formerly Clinical Assistant Professor of Otolaryngology at the University of Illinois College of Medicine. He has published 14 books and more than 400 articles.

the ear itself. When the middle-ear cavity is filled with fluid, it may be necessary to incise the eardrum to induce drainage.

Other Possible Causes

Ear noise is also a symptom of a number of general diseases that indirectly affect the ear through the circulation, as do hypertensive cardiovascular disease and various forms of anemia. It can come, too, from drugs such as quinine and the salicylates, as well as from the excessive and prolonged use of tobacco and alcohol, or, theoretically, from any substance to which the nerve tissue of the auditory mechanism is sensitive.

Working under stress may account for a temporary siege of ear noises, especially in tense, emotional, high-strung individuals besieged by worries, anxieties, and overwork. The noises usually cease when the stress slackens. Finally, head injuries, intracranial tumors, and some diseases of the central nervous system that involve the auditory nerve are additional contributing factors.

Determining the Cause

The effective treatment of ear noise lies, of course, in the removal or treatment of its cause. However, from this brief consideration one can see that it is a symptom of a large number of clinical entities, not all of them related to the auditory apparatus by any means. So it is especially important to examine closely the occasions, events, and conditions surrounding the noise for clues to the cause and guides to proper treatment.

TABLE 1 – MAIN CAUSES OF EAR NOISES

EAR DISORDERS	GENERAL DISEASES
nerve deafness	certain anemias
otosclerosis	hypertensive cardiovascular disease
Ménière's disease	allergy
	respiratory infection
obstruction of eustachian tube	OTHER CONDITIONS
otitis media	certain drugs
irritation of cochlear mechanism	excessive use of tobacco, alcohol
excessive cerumen or cerumen swollen by water in ear	emotional stress
	head injuries
	intracranial tumors
infection	central nervous system diseases involving auditory nerve
fluid in middle ear	

Recently I examined a young high school girl who awoke one morning to find her ear canals itching intensely and her lips and cheeks swollen. She was particularly distressed by the onset of ear noises. The finger of suspicion quickly turned to a dish of sea food that she had eaten the night before. Antihistamines gave prompt relief. Now she excludes oysters, lobsters, and shrimps from her diet.

While looking for clues that will lead to effective treatment, the physician has got to maintain the impression that he understands the seriousness of the annoyance and that he is doing everything possible to help. He must, in other words, try to provide symptomatic relief while looking for the cause.

Not so long ago a tense, high-strung businessman came to me complaining of ear noises that occurred every time he contracted some of the muscles around the ear, face, and jaw. When he was working under pressure, the ear noises intensified, but as soon as the pressure lessened, they stopped. When the patient was assured that the ear noises were the result of anxiety and muscle contractions, he felt greatly relieved that his troubles were not permanent.

What Drugs Are Helpful?

There are many drugs that provide some symptomatic relief to some patients. None has been universally satisfactory, yet each has done some good, and the same can be said for various surgical procedures. Among the drugs that have been found to provide relief occasionally are ephedrine, antihistamines, atropine, calcium, and large oral doses of vitamin B. Iodides and various endocrine preparations are sometimes useful, and so are vasodilators like nicotinic acid. Histamine desensitization seems to help some patients who show a positive response to histamine skin tests. But barbiturates and tranquilizers do the most good symptomatically, especially when administered at night, for ear noise is most disquieting in peaceful surroundings.

Distraction Sometimes Helps

Ear noise usually responds to removal of the underlying cause or to symptomatic treatment, or else it stops spontaneously. However, it sometimes does not. When that happens, preoccupation with some absorbing interest or hobby often provides an antidote. Before bedtime, background music supplied by a radio through earphones may eliminate ear noises from consciousness before the victim falls asleep. The most satisfactory clinical responses are obtained by convincing the patient that everything possible is being done for him, while encouraging him to ignore the ear noises as much as possible.

RELENTLESS FATIGUE
Perhaps Psychogenic?

Fatigue is a normal experience; everybody knows that — including your tired patient. Why then is he asking you to cure it? Obviously, because he believes that something *must* be wrong with anybody who has felt as tired as he has for as long as he has. He may believe he is physically ill, but he probably isn't — not if fatigue is his only symptom. The cause could be environmental, but again it probably isn't. Living in a monotonous, unchallenging, unrewarding, or otherwise unpleasant environment can cause fatigue, and occasionally the environment is inescapable. Usually, though, emotionally mature, intelligent people find ways to modify or escape from unpleasant environments without seeking medical advice. So, common sense leads me to believe that the cause of chronic fatigue is the patient's emotional problems rather than physical illness or environmental problems.

Emotional Causes of Fatigue

To simplify diagnosis, let me list five kinds of patients we are dealing with. In actual practice, they blend to give a great variety of tired patients. (1) The essentially "normal" person in a stressful situation from which he sees no honorable escape. (2) The inadequate person who cannot cope with common life situations. (3) The person who is continually fighting down the impulse to act in some way that he considers immoral or unsocial. (4) The person whose fatigue is a symptom of frank neurosis probably accompanied by anxiety and, in more severe cases, phobias and compulsions. (5) The person whose fatigue is a symptom of depression or a psychosis such as chronic brain syndrome and arteriosclerotic brain disease.

Pitfalls to Avoid in Diagnosis

1. *Paying no attention to fatigue* after the patient complains about it. Fatigue is always a sign that something is wrong, and you ought to find out what it is.

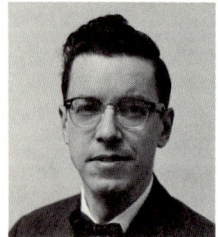

James R. Harris, M.D.
University of Pennsylvania

Doctor Harris is Executive Medical Officer of the Institute of the Hospital of Pennsylvania, and Associate Professor of Psychiatry at the University of Pennsylvania School of Medicine. He is psychiatrist and a trustee at Horizon House (Philadelphia), a rehabilitation center for former mental patients. He is certified by the National Board of Psychiatry and Neurology and is a Fellow of the American Psychiatric Association.

2. *Waiting to ask about possible emotional causes* of fatigue until the physical examination is complete and the results of the laboratory tests are in. This is inefficient since fatigue is more often due to emotional causes than to physical ones. In one group of 235 patients who sought treatment for fatigue, 85% had no detectable physical disease. Worse yet, it misleads the patient. He is likely to think, "The doctor hasn't been able to find the real cause, so now he tells me it's all in my head." Instead he should realize that from the start you are looking for emotional *and* physical causes.

3. *Attributing prolonged, severe fatigue to some transient or trivial physical cause.* This damaging mistake is encouraged by the oft-repeated warning to "rule out physical disease." The implication is that, if physical disease is there, it must have caused the symptoms. Nonsense, of course. If you look hard enough, you can usually find something physically wrong — a low-grade infection perhaps, or a mild anemia that could possibly account for fatigue. Merely mentioning a physical defect is often enough to reinforce the patient's hypochondriasis and divert his attention from the real problem.

4. *Failing to look for signs of depression.* Let me emphasize the common symptoms of depression. In addition to fatigue, they are depressed mood, despair, loss of appetite, insomnia, and a slowing of thought and motion. To assess the possibility of suicide, you need to estimate the depth of the depression. If the patient or someone in his family has attempted suicide before, or if he is extremely restless or sleepless or feels profoundly guilty, suspect suicidal depression.

Questions That Uncover Emotional Causes

Obviously, taking a careful history is essential if you are ever to understand why your patient is tired. Moreover, a good history has therapeutic as well as diagnostic value. By answering questions, your patient is led to a better understanding of himself. I find these questions useful in uncovering the emotional causes of fatigue.

"When are you tired?"

Patients often say, "I'm tired all the time;" this is rarely true. At least, they are much more tired at certain times than at others. Knowing *when* they are most tired may help you to know *why* they are tired. A man may say that he is most tired when he gets home from work at night and that he is not tired on his frequent weekend hunting or fishing trips. There must be something in his home that he is tired of returning to and that he likes to spend weekends away from; you do not need a Sherlock Holmes to single out the wife as a prime suspect. Even more common is the reverse: the inadequate clerk who is "bushed" at 9 a.m. and "rarin' to go" at 5 p.m.

"What relieves the tired feeling?"

Some kinds of emotional fatigue are remarkably easy to relieve — at least, temporarily — by any diversion. For example, a housewife, bedridden by fatigue, somehow found strength to leap from her bed and rearrange newly delivered furniture. When the novelty of the new furniture wore off, her fatigue took possession of her again.

"What do you do all day?"

Even more significant than what the patient does is his attitude toward his activities. Does he derive satisfaction from them? Is the job interesting, difficult, rewarding, worthwhile? Feeling tired has a good deal to do with our interest in what we are doing. In one experiment an athlete in top condition was asked to imitate exactly the movements of a child; after only a few hours he was exhausted. We can surmise that he had lost interest in what he was doing.

"What are your hopes and aspirations?"

Motivation is the antidote of fatigue, both emotional and physical. Overworked physicians who like what they are doing seldom complain seriously about fatigue. On the other hand, we have the tired housewife who, according to a hundred magazine articles, gains no recognition or intellectual stimulation from homemaking. Ask with male logic, "What could be more creative than motherhood, more worthy than molding the future citizens," and she says she would rather do social work or whatever she trained in school to do.

"What could you do if you were not tired?"

For some neurotic patients, fatigue excuses withdrawal from unwanted duties or involvements. A shy person may use fatigue to excuse avoidance of social gatherings. Sometimes it controls an unsocial impulse: nowadays wife-beating is frowned upon, so a hostile husband may suppress his wish to do so with the feeling that his muscles are "paralyzed" by fatigue.

RELENTLESS FATIGUE
Perhaps Organic?

With all due respect to psychiatrists and contemporary teaching, I feel we are twisting the meaning of *psychosomatic* disorder for too many of our tired patients; too often the *psyche* is emphasized at the expense of the treatable *soma*. While there is no question that boredom, loneliness, worry, conflicts, and frustration can exaggerate a sense of total exhaustion, these contributory factors should not overshadow basic organic causes. When your patient's only complaint is "fatigue" that has been present for more than 6 months, make sure the trouble is not basically due to deranged physiology or actual pathology before you label it as psychogenic.

Searching for an organic cause of chronic fatigue may pose a dilemma — either risking diagnostic short cuts on the one hand, or putting your patient "through the mill" of an exhaustive series of X-rays and laboratory tests. Not liking either horn of the dilemma, I pursue the following method for diagnosis. I take a complete history and do a thorough physical examination, keeping in mind the possible organic causes of fatigue (see Table 1). I then arrive at one or several tentative diagnoses and order only those laboratory tests or X-rays necessary to verify or disprove them.

In Table 1, I have listed only the more common "organic" causes of prolonged (arbitrarily 6 months or longer) and unexplained fatigue, italicizing those that experience reminds me warrant the greatest emphasis. I shall not attempt to consider them comprehensively. Obviously, patients with serious infections, hematologic disorders, neoplasms, connective-tissue disorders, and disorders of the central nervous system, peripheral nervous system or musculature will usually have other symptoms besides chronic fatigue.

The All-Important History

In my opinion, *the greatest fault in diagnosing chronically fatigued patients is lack of good history* — that is, failure to clarify what the patient actually means by "fatigue." In this connection, the following

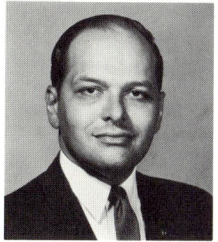

Hyman J. Roberts, M.D.
West Palm Beach, Florida

Doctor Roberts is a former Research Fellow and Instructor in Medicine at the Tufts University and Georgetown Medical Schools. He currently is on the Consulting Staff of Good Samaritan Hospital and St. Mary's Hospital in West Palm Beach, Florida. He is a Diplomate of the American Board of Internal Medicine, a Fellow of the American College of Chest Physicians, and an Associate of the American College of Physicians.

TABLE 1 — CHECK-LIST OF POSSIBLE ORGANIC CAUSES OF CHRONIC FATIGUE

(Italics indicate disorders most frequently found.)

METABOLIC DISORDERS
"Functional" hyperinsulinism
Diabetes mellitus ("diabetogenic hyperinsulinism")
Malabsorption (primary, secondary)
Malnutrition (protein or vitamin deficiency, or both)
Azotemia (chronic renal disease, unrecognized prostatism)
Chronic liver disease (noninfectious)
Intoxications (vitamin A, vitamin D, bromism, alcoholism)

MYOPATHIES
Myasthenia gravis
Periodic paralysis (hypokalemic, hyperkalemic, normokalemic)
Symptomatic myopathies (especially in the granulomatous, connective-tissue, and neoplastic disorders)

SUBACUTE AND CHRONIC INFECTIONS
Hepatitis
Renal-tract infection
Tuberculosis
Brucellosis
Rheumatic fever
Endocarditis

DISORDERS OF THE CENTRAL NERVOUS SYSTEM
Narcolepsy
"Little strokes"
Epilepsy (including its variants or equivalents)
Multiple sclerosis
Parkinsonism

ENDOCRINOPATHIES
Hypothyroidism (primary, iatrogenic, symptomatic)
Hyperthyroidism (Graves' disease, toxic adenoma)
Adrenal insufficiency (primary, iatrogenic, symptomatic)
Ovarian insufficiency (natural or surgical menopause)
Organic hyperinsulinism
Pheochromocytoma
Primary hyperparathyroidism
Adrenocortical hyperfunction

GRANULOMATOUS AND CONNECTIVE-TISSUE DISORDERS
Rheumatoid arthritis
Sarcoidosis
Systemic lupus erythematosus
Polyarthritis

NEOPLASMS
Carcinoma of the pancreas
Retroperitoneal tumors (especially lymphomas)
Carcinoma of the liver (primary, metastatic)
Carcinoma of the cecum and right colon)
Bronchogenic carcinoma
Carcinoma of the kidney

HEMATOLOGIC DISORDERS
The leukemias and lymphomas
Pernicious anemia
Iron-deficiency anemia
Other causes of anemia (notably gastrointestinal and uterine blood loss)
Multiple myeloma
Sickle-cell anemia and its variants

questions may give valuable clues; if the answer is "yes," I then perform those diagnostic tests considered appropriate for the diseases indicated in parentheses.

"Do you have persistent and unrelenting headaches?" (brain tumor)

"Are you troubled by drenching night sweats?" (tuberculosis, nocturnal hypoglycemia)

"Do you have pain in your joints?", or "Does it hurt to breathe?" (systemic lupus erythematosus, rheumatoid arthritis)

"Do you cough a lot?" (tuberculosis, bronchiectasis, lung tumor)

"Have you had a goiter or thyroid operation?" (hypothyroidism)
"Have you ever taken cortisone-type drugs?" (essential, inflammatory, or iatrogenic adrenal insufficiency)
"After you go to bed, are you subject to nightmares, insomnia, 'restless legs,' or severe leg cramps?" (Any two of these, including drenching night sweats mentioned above, should suggest recurrent hypoglycemia.)
"Have you lost your appetite?" (malnutrition, infection, neoplasm)
"Does your fatigue subside promptly after a meal or a snack?" (recurrent hypoglycemia)
"Do you have frequent or unusually foul-smelling bowel movements?" (primary malabsorption)
"Are there any notorious 'sleepyheads' in your family?" (diabetes mellitus, narcolepsy, thyroid diseases)
"Do you often tend to fall asleep while driving, at a party, or at some other social affair?" (narcolepsy)
"During your menstrual period, do you bleed profusely?" (iron-deficiency anemia)
"After childbirth, did you feel weak for several months?" (If the answer is "yes," and the delivery was accompanied by considerable hemorrhage, I suspect pituitary insufficiency.)

Important Physical Clues

To help pinpoint the cause of chronic fatigue, I look for the following clues. If any are found, I perform appropriate diagnostic tests for the diseases indicated in parentheses.

Drowsiness during the interview (narcolepsy)

Sudden sweating, pallor, hunger, tachycardia, or headache (reactive hypoglycemia)

Drooling and poor personal hygiene in a previously fastidious patient (little strokes)

Unequivocal fever (chronic infection, leukemia, lymphoma or other neoplasm)

Marked weight loss (a number of metabolic, hematologic, and neoplastic disorders)

Evidence of cranial nerve dysfunction with inability to sustain muscular activity (myasthenia gravis)

Marked pallor (pernicious anemia, iron-deficiency anemia, blood loss, and other disorders)

Enlargement of lymph nodes or spleen (hematologic disorders, metastatic malignancy, lymphomas)

Sweating, tachycardia, increasing alertness, goiter, fine tremor, exophthalmos (hyperthyroidism)

Dry skin, puffy facies, goiter, neck scar, delayed tendon reflexes in

both contraction and relaxation (hypothyroidism)
    Hypotension and cutaneous oral pigmentation (adrenal insufficiency)

Helpful Diagnostic Tests

After making a tentative diagnosis based on the history and physical examination, I order selected diagnostic tests to help me arrive at a specific diagnosis. The following are routinely used in the case of the more common organic causes of chronic fatigue listed after each test. The list is, of necessity, incomplete.

Hemoglobin determination, red-blood-cell count, hematocrit — iron-deficiency anemia, pernicious anemia, other hematologic disorders

White-blood-cell count, differential — chronic infection, leukemia

Blood glucose, glucose-tolerance test — diabetes mellitus, adrenal insufficiency, pituitary insufficiency, islet-cell tumor

Butanol-extractable iodine, protein-bound iodine, I^{131} uptake — hyperthyroidism (elevated), hypothyroidism (lowered)

Urinalysis, urine culture — renal-tract infection (suspect tuberculosis if sterile in the presence of persistent pyuria), renal neoplasm

Chest X-rays — pulmonary tuberculosis, lymphoma, sarcoidosis, primary or secondary malignancy, intrathoracic goiter

Frequent Oversight

The most frequent oversight I encounter among patients presenting with chronic "refractory" fatigue is failure to recognize the disorder I have called the "syndrome of narcolepsy and diabetogenic hyperinsulinism." In the past 3 years, I have found a great many such patients who were suffering from unrecognized reactive hypoglycemia (with or without impaired glucose-tolerance) and who met at least five of my seven criteria for narcolepsy. On the basis of this experience, I now question *all* "tired" patients about narcoleptic and hypoglycemia symptoms, and obtain glucose-tolerance tests and electroencephalograms, if indicated. I realize that neurologists insist narcolepsy is rare, but my experience consistently indicates its supposed "rarity" largely reflects diagnostic oversight.

On the basis of a personal experience with more than 260 patients having this syndrome, the following pertinent aspects deserve emphasis: (1) it occurs more frequently in females; (2) it occurs at all ages; (3) approximately three out of four patients are significantly overweight; (4) Negroes and children tend to be afflicted with greatest severity; (5) severe hypoglycemia or impaired glucose-tolerance may be demonstrable *only* by afternoon glucose-tolerance testing; (6) thyroid function is normal in the vast majority; and (7) unequivocal dysrhythmias were found in more than 70% of the 110 patients studied by EEG.

TROUBLE STAYING ON A DIET

Most overweight people *can* lose weight permanently. The fact that they usually do not, and have trouble staying on a diet, has caused some doctors to lose interest in helping them. Just telling them they ought to eat less or handing them some standard diet seldom has a lasting effect. Obviously we have to take a more active approach. The question is, do we?

Let's look at a recent survey of 500 obese people who had all received medical treatment for obesity. It revealed that *not one of the 500 remembered having been placed on a definite long-term diet.* This suggests to us that a good many doctors gave up before they started.

Unfortunately, we have no really new suggestions for achieving permanent weight reduction. We shall merely remind you of some of the ideas that have worked well for us. Besides, more important than what we do is how persistently and insistently we do it.

Motivation, Education, and Diet

Motivation is the key problem, of course. Almost all overweight people want to lose weight, but they balk at giving up forever their comfortable eating habits. So, in our first interview, we try to discover why the patient wants to lose weight. Many are concerned about health, and we can honestly reinforce their concern with medical fact. We keep re-

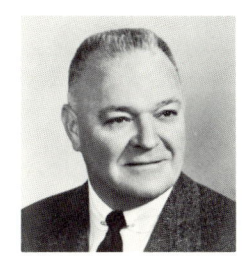

Frank L. Bigsby, M.D.
Chicago, Illinois

Frank L. Bigsby currently is in private practice with Doctor Cayetano Muñiz in Chicago. Doctor Bigsby received his medical education at Tulane University School of Medicine. Before becoming interested in the problems of obesity, he was active in the American Urological Association and was certified by the American Board of Urology in 1943. He served as an officer in the Medical Corps of the United States Army during World War II.

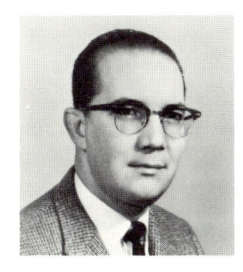

Cayetano Muñiz, M.D.
Chicago, Illinois

Cayetano Muñiz, a graduate from the Havana University School of Medicine, was licensed to practice in Illinois in 1953. Doctor Muñiz served in the Medical Corps of the United States Army during the Korean War. He is presently in private practice with Doctor Bigsby in Chicago. Together they have written a book, PRACTICAL MANAGEMENT OF THE OBESE PATIENT, and five articles on obesity.

minding them that only permanent weight loss can benefit health. Unfortunately, merely recognizing the dangers of obesity is not always enough to keep people slim; if it were we would never see an obese physician.

Vanity is often an even stronger motivating force, and it sometimes provides lasting motivation for socially active, clothes-conscious women. A few people are powerfully and permanently motivated by having a job that depends upon maintaining an attractively slim figure.

Wanting to become slim for special occasions, a vacation or a wedding, for example, is a poor reason for dieting because motivation disappears when the occasion has passed. Even weaker is the motivation that comes from someone else in the family. A good example is the adolescent who sees no compelling reason to curb his appetite although his parents urge him to; you may as well wait a few years until interest in the other sex makes *him* concerned about his appearance.

Naturally we do everything we can to strengthen and preserve each patient's will to reduce permanently. Mainly, we warn of the health hazards of obesity, but we realize that patients' responses are emotional as well as rational. They want our respect and approval and will work to gain them. In fact, most patients need the extra stimulus provided by regular check-up to remain faithful to a diet, just as most of us needed the stimulus of class attendance to learn very much from an anatomy textbook.

Educating patients about weight control ought to be easy but it is not. They need only understand that weight gain and loss result from the difference between the energy derived from food and that used up by working muscles. So simple yet so confining. Little wonder that patients look for exceptions. We repeatedly have to remind them body-fluid fluctuations may obscure loss of fat but only temporarily, that endocrine-caused obesity is rare — so rare, in fact, that Dr. Edward H. Rynearson once remarked, "The only glands involved in obesity are the salivary glands."

When the body expends about 1,500 calories more than it takes in, it withdraws 1 pound of fat from its stores. Hence, in theory, people can reduce by either exercise or diet. In practice, however, we concentrate on diet because we find it easier to induce a patient to routinely refrain from eating a 270-calorie piece of custard pie, for example, than to routinely walk the extra 3 miles needed to burn 270 calories.

Explaining long-term dieting is also difficult. To counter the natural preference for spectacular weight reduction brought about by one magnificent display of self-denial, we now refuse to discuss any goal but gradual reduction over months and years. We begin talking about it at the very first office visit. We tell patients we expect no more than an average weight loss of 5 pounds per month. Since this is an average, they need not be too discouraged later on if they lose only 2 pounds in one month. Indeed, we repeatedly tell our patients that the long-term downward trend has the only really important influence on their health. To focus patients' attention more strongly on long-range view, we forbid them to weigh themselves at home. We advise them to measure their waistlines instead. This gives them some sense of accomplishment, especially at first when loss of fatty tissue may be accompanied by fluid retention resulting in static weight (or even gain) but in smaller girth.

Sensible Diets for the Long Run

Diets for gradual weight loss need not be extreme; many patients will lose weight eating as much as 1,300 or 1,400 calories daily. Before giving specific instruction, we try to get a clear idea of our patients' activities and previous eating habits. If they are fairly active and are eating well-balanced meals, they may be able to lose weight simply by reducing each helping at mealtime by one-fourth and by eliminating snacks. But many others need specific diets that both limit caloric intake and insure good nutrition. We advise patients not to skip meals. We try to restore balance to their diets by allowing some fats and by insisting on sufficient protein. We try to include reduced quantities of as many of the patient's favorite foods as we can. We avoid unreasonable demands that would necessitate two separate menus for the family. We provide for last-minute substitution when he eats out. We urge patients not to eat between meals; for those who find this unbearable we allow snacks of proteins only: meat, poultry products, and sea food but no bread or crackers. We ask them to limit all liquids to 8 glasses per day but do not restrict salt, unless there is some medical reason for doing so.

The object of this program is obvious: we do not think of this diet as a temporary treatment but the basis for future eating habits. Once a patient reaches his natural weight (usually his weight during his early 20's) he is allowed to increase his caloric intake gradually, but we still see him occasionally during the next three years to see that his new habits are firmly established.

By conscientiously applying these ideas to our practice, we have achieved some success in permanent weight reduction. We admit that we can rarely help some kinds of patients — the gourmet, the compulsive eater, the low-calorie metabolizer. But these uncooperative patients seem more common than they are because they go from doctor to doctor looking for some magic that will take the place of self-denial. They ought not to discourage us in our efforts to permanently cure their more typical fellows who will respond to our abiding concern and firm guidance.

DISORDERS IN CHILDREN THAT OUGHT TO BE NEGLECTED

Do we physicians have to give some form of treatment to every child brought to us? Should we prescribe a medicine just because the family expects it? Most of us would readily answer, "Of course not." And yet, because of our training to relieve illness, it is sometimes difficult to resist pressures to "do something" for our patients. Moreover, there are certain conditions in children that are difficult to assess for need of treatment. Let us look at some of these "borderline" conditions where, more often than not, treatment is really not necessary and, in fact, may do more harm than good (see Table 1).

Developmental Variations

Failure to recognize self-limited variations from normal sometimes leads to unnecessary treatment. The "normal" child shows a wide variation in weight, height, and in reaching the landmarks of physical and mental development. Generally, infants tend to lose their fat, baby-like appearance during the second year of life, and at the same time develop day-to-day swings in appetite. This worries parents because they tend to equate *bigness* both in appetite and weight with good *health* (an attitude, incidentally, that may well lead to obesity in later childhood as the child unconsciously seeks to gain approval by overeating).

The parents' overemphasis on food will only be exaggerated further by a prescription for vitamins and tonics to stimulate the appetite. Here is a classic example of a normal process — temporary reduction in food intake — being treated unnecessarily. Instead of being reassured by the doctor's concern, the parents believe that the child's loss of appetite is important. Further, when the treatment with vitamins and tonics does not produce the desired increase in appetite, the parents may lose confidence in the doctor. When faced with an appetite problem in a healthy child, it is much better to take a few minutes to explain that variations are to be expected; showing the child's position on the percentile tables should reassure parents that the child is, in fact, well and needs no medication.

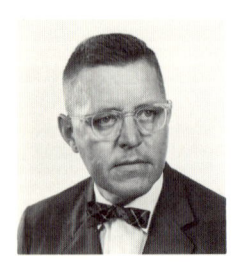

Robert B. Lawson, M.D.
Northwestern University

Doctor Lawson is Chairman of the Department of Pediatrics at Northwestern University Medical School and Chief of Staff of The Children's Memorial Hospital in Chicago. He formerly directed the Department of Pediatrics of the Bowman Gray School of Medicine, and was Chairman of the Department of Pediatrics at the University of Miami School of Medicine.

Minor Defects

Minor defects and variations in development only rarely need treatment, and then only with specific indications. *Umbilical hernia*, even though large, will correct itself without strapping. *Capillary hemangioma*, or port-wine stain, neither goes away nor is satisfactorily treated by any means. *Raised hemangiomas* or strawberry marks will disappear if left alone, and the eventual appearance of the skin is as good as or better than that achieved by treatment which, injudiciously applied, may cause scarring. These lesions usually appear at birth or shortly afterwards, and increase until 7 to 10 months of age. Gradual fading then begins in the center, and the lesions usually disappear by three to five years of age. Many unnecessary *tonsillectomies* are done merely because the tonsils are large; size alone is a poor criterion. There is no evidence that repeated respiratory infections (the most common "reason" for tonsillectomy) are affected by a T & A. *Physiologic flatfoot, bowleg,* and *knock-knee* in the first five years are needlessly treated conditions which are usually completely corrected by the beneficial progress of normal growth. *Tongue-tie* does not create difficulty in nursing and has little if any effect on speech, never causing delay; clipping is indicated only in exceptional cases. *Upper labial frenum* does not cause separation of the incisors and is almost always corrected by eruption of the permanent teeth; surgical removal does not speed up the normal closure. In all these conditions, reassurance and unobtrusive watching will produce a better end-result than ill-advised treatment.

TABLE 1 – SOME DISORDERS IN CHILDREN THAT OUGHT TO BE TREATED WITH INTELLIGENT NEGLECT

Self-limited variations in growth	Bowleg
Temporary poor appetite	Knock-knee
Umbilical hernia	Tongue-tie
Capillary hemangioma	Upper labial frenum
Raised hemangioma	Viral infections of respiratory and gastrointestinal tracts
Enlarged tonsils	
Flatfoot	Functional heart murmur

Viral Infections

Viral infections of the respiratory and gastrointestinal tracts are too often treated with antibiotics. Although these drugs have no antiviral action, the tendency is to use them anyway, either because of fear of missing a bacterial infection, or in order to prevent a complicating bacterial invasion — in spite of the fact that prophylactic therapy has no proven value. It is true that differentiating between viral and bacterial infections is difficult; however, it is not impossible if we consider the clinical picture and the local epidemiologic pattern. When in doubt, we may feel forced to treat, but in doing so should explain why the child is being treated so that undue faith is not built up in antibiotics for viral infections. The excuse that the family demands a shot or a "mycin" does not justify the unwarranted use of potentially harmful and costly drugs.

Problems of Over-Solicitude and Over-Protection

Finally there are situations in which a definite disorder has been diagnosed and probably needs treatment but must be kept in perspective and not exaggerated in importance. A common example in children is the innocent heart murmur. When detected, it should be mentioned to the family but must not be left as a threat to the child. Its innocence must be emphasized, and no restrictions on the child's activities must be allowed. All too often a physician leaves a family in limbo when he says, "We will watch him, but don't let him overdo!" Even if it were an organic murmur, there would be no harm in full activity in the absence of cardiac enlargement or functional impairment. A similar situation follows a diagnosis of rheumatic fever, diabetes, or asthma. Although specific therapy and follow-up prophylaxis are necessary, it is important that as much freedom as possible be allowed in the child's activity so that feelings of inadequacy do not lead to chronic invalidism. Undue restrictions lead only to over-solicitude and over-protection.

A Final Word of Advice

I am saying, in other words, that normal concern and alert observation of a child lead to good preventive measures and healthy guidance, but that over-concern leads to over-treatment. I am not preaching therapeutic nihilism but am urging physicians to recognize those situations where restraint is indicated. There are three such situations: when the treatment may prove more harmful than the disorder itself; when failure to recognize self-limited variations from the normal may lead to insecurity on the part of the parents; and when undue emphasis on treatment may exaggerate the problem it is meant to control.

I know the pressure to "do something" is always there — but often the test of good medicine is to practice the art of intelligent, planned neglect rather than to treat when treatment is not necessary.

SO-CALLED COLIC IN INFANTS

In my opinion, there is no other area of fantasy and fiction comparable in magnitude to that of the well baby care of a newborn infant. High on a list of such errors would be "colic" — because there is a continued belief that colic is a specific disease entity, requiring special treatment and special medicine.

Let's look at some of the facts. If one examined the many thousands of case histories in a large hospital such as Charity Hospital in New Orleans, it is doubtful that any could be found with the primary diagnosis of colic. Yet, how many of us in private practice tell our patients their child has colic? Colic never appears in the hospital newborn nursery; yet, almost immediately after the child's arrival at home, the telephone rings at the doctor's office announcing the appearance of colic.

Colic is practically always found in the first-born; only rarely do parents with two or three children complain that their child has colic. Furthermore, the astute and experienced physician can often foretell by the tension and nervousness of the expectant mother that her child will have colic. These being the facts that attend colic, can one logically conclude that it is an organic disease?

What we call "colic" is not a disease but a problem situation in which both parents and child are adjusting to a new environment. The problem of colic has many causes and predisposing factors: these include a long-accepted folklore, and parental personality factors; most of all, however, the basic problem seems to be a lack of preparation for the responsibilities of parenthood. (Modern society—through the media of television, movies, and books—deceives the prospective parent into expecting an infant who is at all times a restful, lovable, sleeping angel.) Parents are simply not prepared for the day-after-day assault on the nervous system by the crying, straining, struggling, soiled, wet, trembling, hiccuping, bundle of flesh that is man's start on this earth. They are unprepared—emotionally—for the demands that now must be met with personal self-sacrifice to insure their infant's survival.

To make matters worse they are inexperienced, inept, and insecure in their grasp of the day-to-day mechanics of caring for an infant. Their

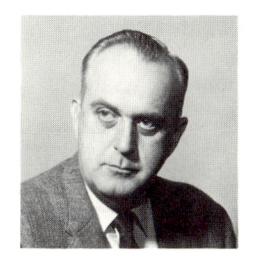

F. Michael Smith, Jr., M.D.
St. Joseph's Hospital, Thibodaux, Louisiana

Doctor Smith, a Fellow of the American Academy of Pediatrics, is Chief of Staff at St. Joseph's Hospital in Thibodaux, Louisiana. He is a past president of the Lafourche Parish Medical Society, and a member of the Louisiana State Medical Society and of the Louisiana State Pediatric Society. His investigative interest lies mainly in pediatric cardiology, and he serves on the Board of Directors of the Louisiana State Heart Association.

insecurity is especially evident when the baby cries, because to them, every cry signals an emergency and inspires panic. Actually, not all crying is due to pain or gastrointestinal dysfunction. It can have as many meanings as the infant has needs, wants, and reactions. Only think of the loud wail you can stimulate by thumping your finger against the sole of the child's foot and you will realize the normal infant's extreme reactivity to his environment. Loud noises, tight clothing, soiled diapers, and, of course, hunger, will cause a normal infant to cry lustily, loud, and long. Also, many infants cry seeking only human contact, pleasant and harmonious sounds, the warmth and security of being held.

The Language of Crying

It is possible for the seasoned parent to detect numerous variations in the way an infant cries which can be understood almost as readily as language. The experienced parent can tell with reasonable accuracy a cry of hunger from a cranky cry, a cry of bearable discomfort from a lonesome cry, and all kinds, unerringly, from the cry of real distress or pain. Unfortunately, such understanding of the infant's piercing attempts at communication is slowly and painfully learned. In the meantime, panic or impatience leads to uncertain, inconsistent handling and so to an uncertain, often crying infant. Quite understandably, parents feel frustrated and inadequate and long for a pat solution to their responsibilities. They are easy prey, at this time, to the recurring suggestion from relatives and friends that their child has "colic."

So, they consult their physician and seek from him a bottle of "colic medicine"—the magic remedy for all their discomfort. To their chronic misfortune, the harrassed physician too often encourages this error—blocking an intelligent appraisal of the child's crying, and beginning a cycle of problems. Soon the medicine is found ineffective. So, formulae are changed and changed and changed. New medicines are endlessly tried, red drops are substituted for green ones, until time and the infant's maturation eventually solve the problem.

There are many reasons for crying and excessive irritability in the newborn but only rarely do they involve organic disease; of course, all such infants merit careful and complete histories and physical examination. For example, some infants manifest gastrointestinal allergy; in these, a trial of 7 to 10 days on hypoallergic formula will act both as a therapeutic and diagnostic measure. Once organic causes have been ruled out, the physician should direct his attention to helping the parents overcome their susceptibility to the colic myth. Here is a method I have found effective in dealing with parents of healthy but "colicky" infants:

• Take a little time to assure the parents that their infant has no disease.

- Explain that crying is the infant's normal means of communication; encourage the parents to listen to it with patience and intelligence.
- Convince them that they are perfectly capable of caring for their child without the help of friends, relatives, and neighbors.
- Teach them a sensible method of feeding the infant.

Overcoming Feeding Problems

The normal newborn takes frequent small feedings of 1 to 2 ounces and desires to nurse at short intervals of one to two hours, taking as many as 10 to 14 bottles in a 24-hour period. To avoid such frequent feedings, parents often thicken the formula, hoping that the child will be satisfied longer and so require less care. Nothing could be farther from the truth. The best artificial formula is one which approaches the isolevel of mother's milk; to thicken the formula beyond this level produces a metabolic stress on the infant — including his intestinal tract, liver, and kidneys. So, many of the irritable, fussy, so-called colic babies are the result of poor formula construction. Subclinical cases of tetany actually exist in children because of hyperelectrolyte mineral load in unaltered cow's milk feeding.

Then, too, there is the question of solid foods. Once it was only with difficulty that parents could be induced to add solid food to the diet of infants. Today, I am alarmed to find what some parents are feeding 2- and 3-week-old infants. Just as there is a normal maturation process for development of neuromuscular achievements, there is a maturation of gastrointestinal function and its readiness to accept solid food. Too early introduction of complex food products can produce irritability and crying in the young infant.

Finally, parents must be encouraged to be flexible in the following of a feeding schedule—feeding the child as much or as little as he desires, as often or as seldom as he desires. Many infants will nurse 3 to 4 ounces of a formula only to awake screaming ten minutes later. When offered another feeding at this time, the child will take only ½ to 1 ounce and fall asleep again for four to six hours. To ignore such variations and adhere rigidly to a clock schedule will result in an irritable, screaming baby until the next bottle is due. Remind the parents, too, that there is no sin in taking an infant in the arms, rocking him, and softly singing a lullaby; this has cured more colic than all the "green drops" in the world.

With an understanding by parents that crying is a normal expression of an infant's desires and reactions, with intelligent feeding, with assurance to parents that they are capable of caring for their infant, with intelligent and loving care, we can eliminate forever the fantasy and fiction that colic is an organic entity.

QUESTIONS AND ANSWERS

Q. What about the infant who screams in apparent agony for an hour or so but when given an enema has immediate relief and falls asleep? Is this not a disease state?

A. This fairly common condition is air-swallowing. Air, which is found in large amounts throughout the infant's gastrointestinal tract, is not due to maldigestion of food. In all instances, any appreciable amount of air is *swallowed* air. This is best prevented by instructing the parent as to "burping" the baby. Sometimes, however, no amount of "burping" will totally prevent air being swallowed and trapped in the bowel to cause distention and discomfort. When this occurs, it is best managed with hot water bottles to the abdomen and, if necessary, a rectal flush.

Q. What about the infant who is tense, screams out without apparent cause, and has hyperactive reflexes? Can this be cured by telling these parents there is no such disease as colic?

A. Obviously the answer is no. The above described infant has an abnormality which is often called the "hypertonic syndrome." This is a separate disorder that must be removed from the "colic" wastebasket grouping. This condition is usually hereditary. A careful history will usually reveal that one or both parents were themselves or that their brothers or sisters were hypertonic children. On examination one finds a tense, jittery infant with hyperactive reflexes. These infants are a trying problem to parent and doctor alike. We have tried all types of sedatives and tranquilizers on them to no avail. One can only reassure the parents that they have a normal healthy baby and that in due time he will outgrow this condition.

Q. What is the ideal formula for an infant?

A. The ideal feeding is of course breast milk. It is indeed unfortunate that in our society, breast feeding is not in current vogue. An attempt at artificial feeding can best be done by imitation of breast feeding. The caloric strength of breast milk is 20 calories per ounce. Thus our formula should be 20 calories per ounce. The protein-fat-carbohydrate ratio of the artificial formula should approach as nearly as possible the same as breast milk. Formulae should not be varied in strength with age or apparent hunger, because nature has not seen fit to do so with breast milk.

ALLEGED GROWTH PROBLEMS IN CHILDREN

If there were a completely normal child, he would be such a rarity that he could not justifiably be called "normal." Consider, for example, the variations in "normal" *growth* of children. If you look at three healthy 4-year-olds, one might be 44 inches tall and weigh 49 lbs. (large-normal, 97th percentile); another, the so-called average child, might be 41 inches tall and weigh 36 lbs.; and the third, only 38 inches tall and 29 lbs. (small-normal, 3rd percentile). All three children would be "normal"; yet the difference in height and weight between the largest and the smallest is 6 inches and 20 lbs. This wide range of "normal" is important for us to keep in mind and to make clear to parents of young children. When we do not, the children are often subjected to parental concern that can produce symptoms and even evoke wrong diagnoses and inappropriate treatment.

Children Who Are "Too Small"

Recently, we surveyed records of visits to a private pediatric office to see how many parents were worried about the growth and development of their children. *In one visit out of every five, the mother expressed concern about her child's growth.* Usually, she was worried that her child was "too small" for his age; this was especially true for boys between two and five years old, a period when normal children are relatively thin and growth is slow (see Figure 1). Actually, all of these "too small" children were within normal range and many were truly average in weight and height.

Why, then, should these parents have been so worried about healthy children? In preschool children, the most important reason is that parents are unprepared for the change from the permissive, rapidly growing baby with high caloric needs into a resistant, slowly growing, thin child with low caloric needs. This change usually occurs when the child first uses his highchair to become a member of the family circle at mealtime. The small newcomer gets a plate just like Dad's, portions of food that are similarly too large, and an ultimatum to eat every bite.

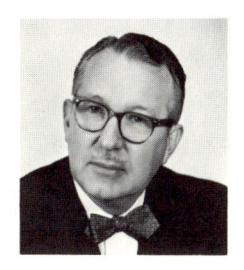

James L. Dennis, M.D.
University of Arkansas

Doctor Dennis is Associate Dean and Professor of Pediatrics at the University of Arkansas Medical Center. He is also an official examiner for the American Board of Pediatrics; Fellow, American Academy of Pediatrics; Secretary, Section on Pediatrics, American Medical Association; and member of the Southern Society for Pediatric Research.

"nuisance" complaints

With so much attention focused on the amount of food he consumes, he is almost certain to lose more of his already small appetite. So, the battle of the dinner table begins.

There's an old joke about "pediatricians eating because Johnny doesn't." Unfortunately, the battle of the dinner table is no joke. Because the preschool years are formative ones that lay the foundation for a sound viewpoint about one's self and one's place in this world, this battle can leave permanent scars. What happens to the basic security of a normal little boy whose anxious, well-meaning mother alternates between mealtime nagging and forced feedings? What if his father obviously wishes for a more manly-looking boy and appears to deny him approval and acceptance because of what he is — a small boy? His parents may even compare him unfavorably to a heavier brother or sister and make him feel guilty and somehow less lovable because he is thin. Sometimes, the physician unwittingly joins the battle by prescribing everything from tonics to androgenic hormones in a misguided effort to produce a "super-normal" boy. When this happens, the boy can really be sure that he is a problem and a disappointment to his parents. He is sure to have difficulty in developing confidence in himself, and may be plagued by self-doubt for the rest of his life.

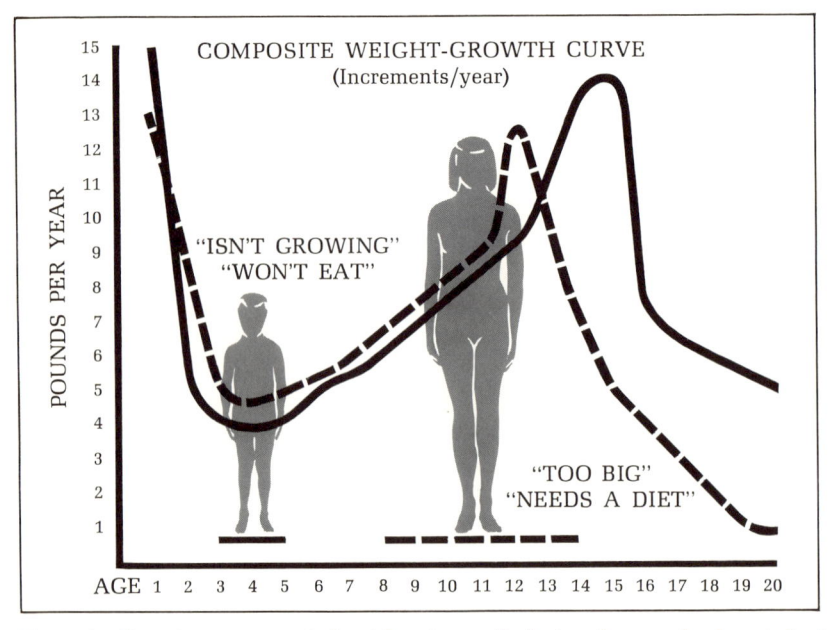

Figure 1 — Parents worry most about boys' growth during the preschool period of minimal growth; about girls', during maximal growth of adolescence.

Children Who Are "Too Large"

Concern about children who are "too large" is much less common; but it does occur, almost exclusively in parents of girls between the ages of nine and 14. Girls of this age commonly experience a spurt in height for which their parents are unprepared and which alarms both the parents and the girls themselves. This alarm is understandable when you realize that the possible normal spread in height and weight for 12-year-old girls may be as much as 12 inches and 64 pounds. The worry is often complicated, too, by the fact that large girls mature early.

What about the 97th percentile girl who is taller than all the boys in her class and whose large mother tearfully recalls her own distressing adolescence? This child really has a problem, but it is not one that requires or even justifies hormonal intervention. Unfortunately, there is a current trend today toward trying to close the epiphyses with estrogen therapy. To me, such therapy seems unwise and wholly unjustified. We have seen some pre-adolescent girls who developed premature menarche as a result. Aside from the fact that we do not know what the long-range effects of such therapy may be, we are not even sure that it produces the desired effect on height. In most instances, estrogen therapy stimulates a period of very rapid growth before epiphyseal closure; as a result, many of these girls probably end up at the same height they would have attained naturally.

Instead of applying dubious or possibly harmful therapy, we should help these girls to accept themselves for what they are — tall, normal children. If we take the time to give confidence-building reassurance, we can help them realize that tallness can be a tool of leadership and a great asset. One practical way to build self-confidence might be to suggest that they enroll in a charm and grooming course.

What Can We Do?

Whether the child is "too small" or "too large," the most reassuring thing you can do is to plot the child's growth on the percentile grid and use this as a visual aid while talking with the parents and the child.

Instead of allowing parents to pressure you into prescribing unnecessary and possibly dangerous medication, you would do better to prepare parents for the expected changes in growth and development, and to try to find out if they have false beliefs about growth. This takes a little more time initially than the writing of a prescription, but it saves you time in the long run. Here are some points you may find helpful:

• Remember that simple verbal assurance such as "Johnny is normal" is not enough.

• You'll need to let the parents follow his growth by plotting weight and

height on a percentile grid.
- Make sure that *both* parents see the child's growth chart. When you reassure the mother alone, she may fail to transmit this confidence to the father and he may continue to think that his child is being neglected.
- Try to anticipate growth problems by explaining to parents just what they should expect of the child, especially at problem stages of development. These problem stages are most apt to occur in boys during the preschool period of smallest growth and in girls during the adolescent period of greatest growth.

Comment

Most "growth problems" in children are not medical problems at all, but merely a result of parental misinformation on what constitutes normal development. If we are going to keep anxious parents from pressuring us into treating normal children for "endocrine" problems, we must be thoroughly familiar with the many variations of normal development and always keep these variations in mind.

chapter 2

COMPLAINTS ABOUT THE RESPIRATORY SYSTEM

MANY-FACED ASTHMA

Asthma is not, in itself, a diagnosis. Instead, it is the manifestation of any disease in which diffuse ventilatory obstruction produces bothersome symptoms. The causes are specific only on occasion. More often, they are multiple; most often, they are simply not known.

When the pathogenesis of any disease is complex or unknown, it is tempting for one to become a diagnostic "splitter" rather than a "lumper." If I were to yield completely to this temptation, I would end up discussing eight or nine different forms of diffuse obstructive lung disease. Instead, I will discuss three main groups because they offer the greatest challenge to differential diagnosis and treatment. These are *atopic asthma, nonatopic asthma,* and *chronic obstructive pulmonary emphysema.* All three have one feature in common: they are diffuse pulmonary diseases with obstruction to expiratory air flow. This obstruction occurs because of varying combinations of bronchospasm, mucosal edema, intrabronchial secretions, interstitial inflammation, basement-membrane thickening, vasodilation, and fibrosis. The relative proportion of each varies with pathogenesis and influences the response to therapy. Emphysema itself, due mostly to air trapped in alveoli behind the bronchiolar obstruction, is of secondary importance and is potentially reversible, in the first two groups. In chronic obstructive emphysema, by contrast, the emphysema is related to loss of alveolar structure, and much of the obstruction is due to diminished elastic support of the bronchioles; they tend to collapse on expiration. Little can be done to reverse these defects.

Proper classification of asthma requires the use of relatively simple clinical and laboratory clues that are often overlooked. One should look for sputum and blood eosinophilia and get a quantitative recording of the expiratory flow rate. Skin tests may be necessary if specific allergic sensitivity is suspected from the history. In general, such tests should include *common* environmental allergens likely to be inhaled, such as feathers, animal danders, house dust, and those pollens and molds appropriate to the history and the region.

Here is more about the three broad types of obstructive lung disease.

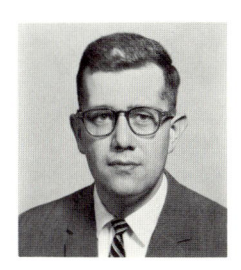

Paul P. VanArsdel, Jr., M.D.
University of Washington

Doctor VanArsdel is Associate Professor of Medicine and Head of the Division of Allergy at the University of Washington School of Medicine. He is President-Elect of the Washington State Allergy Society, and a Fellow of the American Academy of Allergy and of the American College of Physicians. His research efforts have focused mainly on histamine metabolism, drug allergy, and mechanisms of human allergic reactions.

Atopic Asthma

Atopic asthma is characterized by the hereditary tendency to develop circulating skin-sensitizing antibodies to foreign substances that are generally innocuous to man. The most frequent disorders of atopic patients are infantile eczema, hay fever, and asthma. Most have some difficulty before the age of 30. Atopic asthma is paroxysmal; the severity of the attacks depends on the amount of inhaled allergens. Moderate blood eosinophilia — from 400 to 1,000 cells per cu. mm. — is found during symptomatic periods. The vital capacity may be low with a slow expiratory flow rate even in the absence of symptoms, but should return to normal within minutes after administration of epinephrine subcutaneously or use of a nebulized bronchodilator. Skin testing usually produces strong whealing reactions, particularly to pollens, and should be done cautiously, starting with scratch tests, or intradermal tests using weak solutions. Asthma that appears in the spring or early summer is most likely caused by pollens. If the asthma is worse in late summer and early fall, weed pollen or mold spore sensitivity should be suspected. Winter asthma is likely to be associated with household allergens such as dust or feathers. Occasionally, questionable allergy can be confirmed or ruled out by having the patient inhale the suspected antigen and checking the change in vital capacity.

Nonatopic Asthma

Nonatopic asthma (or *intrinsic* asthma) characteristically starts after the age of 30, sometimes without personal or familial allergic history. It is often associated with chronic infection, particularly of the paranasal sinuses. Affected patients may have nasal or sinus polyps and some have an unusual sensitivity to aspirin. Many blood and sputum eosinophiles are often present, generally more than in uncomplicated atopic asthma. The vital capacity and flow rate are affected as in atopic asthma, but impairment is more pronounced. Improvement with bronchodilators is usually incomplete. Adrenocortical steroid therapy may be required for optimal improvement. Except for occasional moderate reactions, skin tests are negative. Although bacterial allergy is often suspected in these patients, skin tests for bacterial antigens are unreliable and proof of bacterial allergy is difficult to get.

Obstructive Pulmonary Emphysema

Obstructive pulmonary emphysema has a natural history quite different from asthma; it is often confused with asthma. It rarely becomes symptomatic before the age of 40. While there is no allergic history, this condition may be preceded by several years of chronic cough or recurrent respiratory infections. The patients usually have a history of heavy cigarette smoking or prolonged exposure to industrial air pollution. Usually gradually and relentlessly progressive with no asymptomatic periods, it often gets much worse when the patient picks up a minor respiratory infection. There is no blood eosinophilia and sputum eosinophiles are scanty. The vital capacity may be low or normal, but the ventilatory flow rate is always slow. In contrast to the true asthmatic, who can expire for only three or four seconds, a patient with this disorder may require up to 12 seconds to achieve his full vital capacity. Although the patient may feel better, the timed vital capacity is not improved to any great degree by treatment. Bronchodilators may effect 5% to 10% improvement at best; adrenocortical steroids seem to have no specific effect whatsoever. Skin tests for antigens are negative.

These three disorders are not distinct. True asthmatics may develop irreversible obstructive changes with chronic inflammation and fibrosis; they do not develop the fenestration and loss of alveolar septa characteristic of obstructive emphysema. Chronic bronchitis may lead to peribronchial inflammation and fibrosis, with the diffuse obstructive symptoms, but not the reversibility, of asthma. Some asthmatics develop such chronic, irreversible changes.

Some atopic asthmatic patients may develop a more persistent and complicated disease with associated chronic infection and more eosinophilia, and control of allergic factors is no longer adequate.

"Asthmatic bronchitis" is a term that is used indiscriminately in many different contexts, but it is probably a real entity in the young child who develops wheezing during acute respiratory infections and has no subsequent trouble. This may be very serious, as in the "obstructive bronchiolitis" of infancy. In the older patient, "asthma" appearing with respiratory infections or cardiac failure may reflect underlying obstructive pulmonary disease.

Management

There are significant differences in the management of these disorders:
1. *Environmental control* — Avoiding respiratory irritants may help in all these disorders, but it is most important in obstructive emphysema. Affected patients should stop smoking and avoid polluted atmospheres. The most effective therapy for atopic asthma is eliminating offending antigens inside the home. An effective household filtering system may also provide considerable relief by limiting the influx of pollen and mold spores, and clearing the air of house dust.

Whether to advise patients to move to a "better climate" should depend on the basic disease. Atopic asthmatics are often urged to move to a "dry climate" with unfortunate results. Seasonal pollen asthma in New York or Detroit may turn into perennial pollen asthma in warm, dry, well-irrigated Arizona or California. On the other hand, patients with non-atopic asthma and obstructive emphysema may improve dramatically in such climates. No patient, however, should be advised to move without a trial period in the new area first.

2. *Bronchodilator drugs* — Drugs such as epinephrine or theophylline may help in true asthma, but not much in obstructive emphysema. Patients with this disease may use a remarkable amount of nebulized epinephrine or isopropylarterenol in a desperate attempt to get a minor improvement in ventilatory flow rate. These drugs seem to work only to the degree that mucosal edema is reduced and sputum is mobilized.

3. *Adrenal cortical steroids* — Both atopic and nonatopic asthma may improve dramatically with steroid therapy; this is reflected by marked improvement in vital capacity and ventilatory flow rate. However, in nonatopic asthma particularly, it is difficult to discontinue steroids. Although steroids may give some subjective relief to patients with chronic obstructive emphysema, they do not improve ventilatory function. Steroid treatment is inadvisable for such patients, since the risk of steroid therapy outweighs the minor subjective benefits.

4. *Hyposensitization* — When asthma is related to specific antigens by the history and by immediate skin reactions, hyposensitization of the patient with those antigens is beneficial, but obviously less effective than avoiding the antigens entirely. However, such treatment of nonatopic asthma has little influence on the course of the disease. The patient with obstructive pulmonary emphysema is sometimes given a long series of such injections on the basis of an incorrect diagnosis of asthma and some minor or false positive skin-test reactions. A more physiological approach to therapy for that patient would be far more beneficial.

5. *Supportive measures* — Breathing exercises, postural drainage, sputum liquefiers, intermittent positive-pressure breathing, and antibiotic therapy are helpful for the true asthmatic, particularly during the early phases of management. Good treatment of chronic obstructive emphysema, however, must depend largely on such measures, since bronchodilator drugs are relatively ineffective by themselves, and steroids are of no value.

The role of psychological factors in asthma is often difficult to assess; emotional stress may aggravate asthma in one patient, but relieve it in another. Whether one should do more than provide the strong, sympathetic support which every patient deserves, depends on the individual problems involved. Associated emotional disturbances may require psychotherapy; asthma alone, does not.

NOT-SO-SIMPLE ALLERGY

When a physician says to a patient, "You're allergic," or, "You have an allergy," he is not really making a diagnosis. Until he determines what the patient is allergic *to*, he cannot be certain the patient is allergic at all.

Most allergic symptoms can be mimicked by other disorders. Emotional stress, in particular, often produces symptoms — stuffy nose and urticaria are two — that might wrongly be blamed on some allergen.

Before starting to look for allergens by various tests, the physician should be reasonably certain that allergy exists, and that the symptoms are appropriate for the suspected allergy. This article will discuss some clues that may help confirm a suspicion of allergy, as well as the most significant tests used to pin down the offending allergens.

Clues for Suspecting Allergy

A diagnosis of allergy in some patients can be made reasonably well from the history and physical examination. A history of atopic disease (asthma, hayfever, or eczema) in the patient or his family is helpful, and the pattern of his symptoms can provide important clues.

Complaints which are intermittent or paroxysmal, and related to changes in the environment or to changes in the season of the year, are more likely to be allergic than those which are chronic or which fluctuate with no particular pattern.

The diagnosis of contact eczema and of atopic dermatitis is aided by the appearance and location of the lesions. The bluish-red, swollen nasal mucous membrane is considered classical for nasal allergy, and nasal polyps are rarely, if ever, present in the absence of allergy. Diagnosing allergy in a patient with asthmatic symptoms is more difficult, and the history is often more helpful than the physical signs of diffuse expiratory wheezing, which are common to several disorders.

Allergic fever is uncommon, and should only be considered when other causes of fever have been ruled out.

Standard laboratory tests may be of some help. Eosinophilia is the most helpful finding, if present. The blood eosinophiles are elevated in

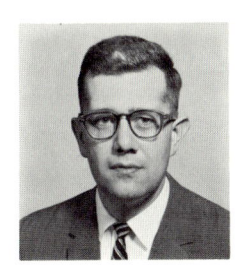

Paul P. VanArsdel, Jr., M.D.
University of Washington

Doctor VanArsdel is Associate Professor of Medicine and Head of the Division of Allergy at the University of Washington School of Medicine. He is President-Elect of the Washington State Allergy Society, and a Fellow of the American Academy of Allergy and of the American College of Physicians. His research efforts have focused mainly on histamine metabolism, drug allergy, and mechanisms of human allergic reactions.

bronchial asthma, and there should be numerous eosinophiles in the sputum. In allergic rhinitis, blood eosinophilia may be absent, but the presence of eosinophiles in the nasal secretions is diagnostic. In dermatitis, blood eosinophilia may develop without demonstrable allergy, so is of less diagnostic value.

It seems to me that neither a low nor high white-blood-cell count is of any real diagnostic value. In my experience, leukopenia is caused only rarely by an allergic state; most patients have normal or slightly elevated counts.

Similarly, serum gamma globulins show no consistent change. Tissue biopsies are indicated only in the more confusing or obscure conditions and the changes are often nonspecific.

Here are brief descriptions of the various tests for allergy.

The Patch Test

The patch test, used to detect a delayed-type sensitivity to contactants, requires little time and equipment. Standard dermatology and allergy texts list the usual offending substances and explain the way to prepare them. One can also buy ready-to-use testing kits. Some substances, such as rubber, can be applied directly to the skin, but others may be primary irritants and should be used with caution.

Patches are best placed on the patient's back, after his skin lesions have largely cleared. The positive reaction is pruritic, erythematous, and usually vesicular. Ordinarily, the patch is kept on for 48 hours; however, the patient should be told to remove it at once if itching and burning starts, to avoid the appearance of an excessive, possibly ulcerative lesion. Occasionally the reaction may not become positive until 72 hours. The patch test, when done properly, is the most specific of all allergy tests.

The Scratch Test

The scratch test, used to detect immediate hypersensitivity, is performed by breaking the surface of the skin by any practical method that does not produce bleeding. Scarifiers can be obtained from companies that supply antigens, but the job can be done just as well with a narrow Bard-Parker blade; I often use a 20-gauge needle. The scratches should be about ¼" long, and placed on the forearm; they should be 1" apart, if possible.

Scratch testing has several advantages for the general physician. The antigens are supplied in concentrated solutions and, if refrigerated, are stable for three years. They can be applied to the scratches rapidly, and the excess can be wiped off if a strong reaction develops. The tests are usually read after 25 minutes and graded either as negative (same as control site), or from 1 plus to 4 plus. The control reaction (to diluent alone) may be marked in some patients; nevertheless, it is the negative against which the severity of other reactions must be judged. In general, a 4-plus reaction should include a central wheal at least 1 cm. in diameter with one or more pseudopods and surrounded by erythema.

Scratch tests have been of most value for detecting pollen sensitivity. I would say, then, that the best investment for the physician interested in testing a few patients is a set of scratch-test antigens for pollens common in his area. This set should include several grasses, three or four weeds, and a half dozen tree pollens; it is most appropriate for testing patients with spring, summer or fall hay fever or asthma. Most people who are sensitive to grass or weed will have strong reactions.

In adults, scratch tests for house dust, feathers, animal danders, fungi, and other inhalant allergens are rarely adequate. I do not use them at all except in the patient whose history shows he's unusually sensitive. Children, however, do react to such antigens, and the pediatrician may find a set of them useful. The important thing to remember is this: *negative scratch tests do not rule out allergy!*

Because scratch tests are less accurate than intradermal tests, many allergy clinics use them only as a screening procedure, to detect a strong sensitivity to allergens. Weak-positive reactions are always checked by intradermal tests, which may then show anything from a negative to a 4-plus reaction! Naturally, antigens that produce 3-plus or 4-plus reactions by the scratch test should not be given intradermally.

Some allergists use puncture tests in place of scratch tests; principles of selection and interpretation are the same as for the scratch tests.

The Intradermal Test

The intradermal test is more specific than the scratch test for detecting immediate hypersensitivity. A tuberculin syringe and short-bevel hypodermic needle are used to inject, intradermally, about 0.02 cc. or less of a sterile dilute antigen solution — enough to produce a 1/16″ bleb.

The injection is best made on the outer aspect of the upper arm. Fifteen minutes later, the reaction is read and graded in the same way as a reaction to the scratch test. The physician who does this test must make certain he injects the proper amount of a properly diluted solution. One of the most common errors in intradermal testing is the use of large volume (0.1 cc.), as if one were doing a tuberculin test. This volume, besides giving false-positive reactions, has probably contributed to fatal systemic reactions. By the way, if a systemic reaction does occur, a tourniquet placed above the testing site (followed by appropriate medication) is the best way to control it. This is one reason to test on the arm, not the back.

Intradermal tests can also be used to detect delayed skin hypersensitivity. In practice, however, this is done only to discover sensitivity to bacterial and fungal antigens, such as tuberculin and histoplasmin. Positive reactions indicate only a previous exposure and not active disease. In particular, tests to determine sensitivity to such bacteria as streptococcus or staphylococcus are of no value in diagnosing bacterial allergy. Many normal people will show positive reactions merely because they have been adequately exposed to these bacteria.

The antigens used in the intradermal test, unlike those used in the scratch test, must be replaced yearly. Keeping a large supply on hand is costly and, for most physicians, not very practical. Those physicians who wish to be set up for limited intradermal testing will find that a high percentage of sensitivities can be detected with the following solutions: house dust, mixed feathers, dog dander, cat dander, mixed fungi, mixed trees, mixed grasses, and mixed weeds.

Blood Tests Usually Not Practical

Specific allergy can be detected by giving the allergic patient's serum intradermally in several sites to a nonallergic volunteer, and then testing those sites. This test requires special facilities and precautions, and is used only by the trained allergist or investigator when an unusual clinical situation exists.

Certain other techniques involving such things as the flocculation of antigen-coated particles, white-cell lysis, and turbidity reactions have been publicized, but experienced investigators have found them worthless. There is as yet no practical method for the detection of specific drug, food or inhalant allergens by laboratory blood or serum tests. The new basophile-degranulation test is still experimental; it seems to have no advantage over skin testing.

Food and Drug Allergies

Skin testing for sensitivity to foods, whatever the technique, often leads to confusion rather than diagnosis, even in the best allergy clinics. Better avoid it, except possibly for scratch tests limited to 5 to 10 selected foods, given to the young child or infant, in whom a positive reaction is more often significant. More extensive testing should be left to the experienced allergist.

Skin tests are not of much value in determining drug sensitivity either — a fact that a surprising number of physicians do not seem to realize. Most drugs are simple chemicals and probably produce sensitivity by combining with proteins in the body. The patch test for contact dermatitis is dependable and specific because it is administered in the same way the drug was used in treatment. Although a systemic drug reaction, such as fever or skin rash, also can be proven by giving the drug again, this can be dangerous. Skin tests are rarely positive in patients with urticaria or other systemic drug allergies except when the drug is of protein origin (ACTH, horse serum and insulin, for example). In a special situation (severe anaphylactic sensitivity), penicillin is another exception.

Certain reactions, such as serum sickness, depend on the appearance of allergy some time *after* a drug or antiserum is given. Obviously, doing a skin test beforehand will not prevent the use of the drug. New approaches, such as the use of penicilloyl polylysine for skin testing for penicillin allergy, may be valuable, but cannot be recommended for general use until expert evaluation is completed. The most important reason for skin testing with antitoxin or penicillin is to detect severe anaphylactic sensitivity and save the patient from a potentially fatal reaction. However, even the skin test can give a bad reaction in such patients, so must be done with caution.

A Principle to Remember

As you can see, then, the "diagnosis" of allergy is incomplete and may even be confusing, unless supported by simple, but carefully selected, methods of getting at the cause. Without the cause, the diagnosis is meaningless, yet we have a long way to go before adequate and safe tests are available for all causes of allergy.

COUGHS AND COUGHING

An old adage avers that there is "nothing so bad for a cough as coughing." It refers, of course, to the "chronic cough," the cough that repeats and repeats, sometimes with an obvious cause, sometimes with a serious hidden cause, sometimes with no apparent cause at all. It isn't always easy to draw the line between the acute and the chronic cough. Take whooping cough, for example: it lasts and lasts for weeks and weeks. But even so, it does have a foreseeable end, whereas a chronic cough may go on for months or years. The question is, what is causing it?

A cough is a momentary closure of the glottis combined with an explosive expiration of air produced by a contracture of the thoracic cage. It is nature's way of removing the cause of an irritation to the sensitive mucosa of the respiratory tract. How sensitive the mucosa is, is quite evident to anyone who has accidentally swallowed water "the wrong way." Chevalier Jackson called this protective cough "the watchdog of the lungs." The patient with a chronic cough begins to feel that his watchdog is overly protective, and so do the people around him.

A chronic cough may vary in intensity from a distressingly severe paroxysm to scarcely perceptible but persistent, even subconscious, urge to "clear the throat," often an almost involuntary reflex without any evident irritation to justify it. The repetitious coughing serves only to aggravate the irritation it is designed to eliminate.

What Is Causing It?

When coughing persists without any apparent cause, a systematic examination is called for. Although it is primarily a pulmonary phenomenon, coughing may result from disorders of the ear, nose, or throat. In examining the ears, look for excessive cerumen or a small foreign body in the external auditory canal; either one can set off vigorous coughing. In examining the nose, look for possible secretions produced by chronic rhinitis or sinusitis, dropping into the sensitive lumen of the larynx and trachea; this is a common cause of chronic cough. In examining the throat and pharynx, look for hypertrophic lymphoid nodules on the pos-

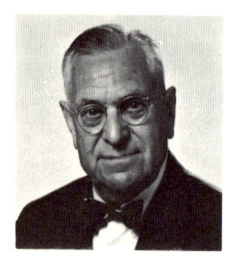

Lyman G. Richards, M.D.
Wellesley Hills, Massachusetts

Doctor Richards is Secretary of the American Laryngological Association. He received his medical education at Harvard Medical School, at St. Luke's Hospital, New York, and at the Massachusetts Eye and Ear Infirmary, Boston. He is a past president of the American Laryngological, Rhinological and Otological Society and also of the American Broncho-Esophagological Association.

terior pharyngeal wall. If present, they may be acting as a source of mucosal irritation and producing the coughing. Obviously, in such cases, coughing only serves to increase the irritation and create a vicious cycle, so treatment must be directed towards eliminating the nodules. Often simply applying 10% silver nitrate to the nodules will diminish or eradicate the irritation. If the irritation persists, you can excise the nodules easily with a ring punch, after first applying a local anesthetic. Nose drops, gargles, lozenges, and similar medications are usually ineffective in such cases, because they fail to reach the mucosa harboring the lymphoid tissue.

Consider the Possibility of Habitual Coughing

Sometimes persistent coughing merges from acute into chronic; the coughing may become a habit. As I mentioned before, whooping cough is perhaps the best example, but even after weeks of persistence, there is a foreseeable end with recovery. Incidentally, though it is essentially a childhood malady, adults may be victims of whooping cough, even as late as the seventh or eighth decade. Indeed, adults may be seriously ill with it.

Sometimes coughing, or throat-clearing, persists long after the cause has been eliminated. Sometimes it persists even when there is no apparent cause. In either case, you are likely to be dealing with a habit, sometimes one with an emotional cause. The habit may be broken with suggestion, but if "psychogenic" cough is a persistent social handicap, you may have to call upon a psychiatrist for help.

Contrary to popular opinion, an elongated or edematous uvula is not a likely source of chronic cough. Although true in a few cases, so many people have this condition without the slightest tendency to coughing that hasty amputation of the uvula is never wise.

Mirror Examination Is Useful

Certain pathological conditions within the larynx itself may cause chronic coughing but may be overlooked unless coughing is coupled with hoarseness. Laryngeal abnormalities such as a pedunculated polyp, a subglottic cyst, a hemangioma, or an unsuspected foreign body can be detected only by a mirror examination.

Lower in the respiratory tract, look for tracheitis. Chronic tracheitis produces a dry hacking cough that may persist for weeks or months, especially in the winter and in excessively dry climates. Although not incapacitating, it may persist in spite of therapeutic steam inhalations. Modern home heating, with its tendency to dry the air, often causes tracheitis, but routine use of a home humidifier may counteract the dryness. Often, tracheitis will not be cured until the patient moves to a warmer or damper climate.

Serious Hidden Causes of Chronic Cough

The three serious causes of chronic cough lie deeper than the larynx, in the lung tissue itself: pulmonary tuberculosis, cancer, and chronic bronchiectasis. Despite giant strides made through public health measures — mass X-ray examinations and publicity — tuberculosis still goes unconquered. To assume that it could not be the cause of a patient's chronic cough is to risk not only the individual patient's health and life, but also that of people with whom he comes in contact. If you detect only a single person with tuberculosis out of 100 coughing patients for whom you have ordered chest X-rays and sputum analyses, all the labor and expense will be justified.

Suspect Lung Cancer

No potential cause of chronic cough is more in the public eye today or of more concern to the medical profession than cancer of the lung. Because a chronic, often unproductive cough may be the earliest and often the only symptom, the possibility of cancer should be kept in mind. Chest X-ray, sputum smears, and bronchoscopy are "musts" to establish or exclude this diagnosis. Radical thoracic surgery has done much to lower the mortality from lung cancer, but this disease still takes entirely too many lives that might have been saved by earlier suspicion of its role in producing a chronic cough.

Smoking, particularly of cigarettes, has also long been considered a cause of chronic coughing by many clinicians. Paradoxically, however, a heavy smoker may never complain of a cough. Most of us are inclined to proscribe all use of tobacco when our patients complain of chronic cough, and this may indeed be the correct solution, but we can never safely assume that some more serious etiology is not involved.

Consider Chronic Bronchiectasis

The third of the pulmonary triad, chronic bronchiectasis, is characterized — perhaps more often than either tuberculosis or lung cancer — by a chronic cough, one that usually is productive of moderate to copious purulent secretion. Again, the only way to make a definite diagnosis is to do a thorough physical examination and order X-rays and sputum studies. As an adjunct to X-ray study, instilling an opaque iodized oil into the tracheobronchial tree will help delineate the bronchial dilatations and sacculations. This enables localizing one or more portions of the lung that may have to be removed surgically. Repetitive bronchoscopic aspiration of secretions, often used to relieve bronchiectasis, can be palliative but will not cure the disease. Therefore, your patients with suspected bronchiectasis should be referred for possible surgery. Incidentally, the technique of introducing an opaque oil into the tracheobronchial tree for X-ray study is not especially difficult for anyone who has acquired reasonable facility in the use of the laryngeal mirror. The larynx and trachea must be anesthetized with a suitable topical agent and the patient must be cautioned not to cough (lest he force oil into the alveoli), and then a curved radiopaque catheter on a removable stylet can be slipped through the larynx under indirect mirror vision and carried to various levels in the tracheobronchial tree. Under immediate fluoroscopic guidance, oil can then be instilled from an attached syringe, and any desired area of the lung can be mapped out and films taken on the spot, before any of the oil can diffuse from the area.

Allergy May Be Causing Cough

Chronic cough may also result from allergy. As in all allergic conditions, the solution to the problem lies in discovering and, if possible, eliminating the offending allergen.

Forgotten Foreign Body

When a patient has a chronic cough with no other apparent cause, suspect the possibility that a small object has somehow become trapped in the bronchial tree. Unless the foreign body is detected by X-ray or bronchoscopic examination, serious and often avoidable pulmonary damage may result. A boyhood friend of mine unknowingly carried a carpet tack in his upper lobe bronchus for years before a physician suggested an X-ray. This resulted in bronchoscopic removal of the tack and complete restoration of my friend's health.

* * *

Most chronic coughs can be diagnosed successfully if you remember to take a complete history, make a thorough examination, and resist the temptation to belittle the cough as "nothing serious."

PERSISTENT COLDS — OR IS IT AN ALLERGY?

"Is it a cold or an allergy?" the patient often asks me. When he does, I turn it around, and I ask *him* a few questions:

"*How often do you have a cold?*"
Ordinarily, a person will have only two or three a year. Repeated and frequent colds ("a cold all the time" or "one cold after another") suggest an allergic reaction.

"*How long do your colds last?*"
If longer than two or three weeks, he probably has a purulent sinusitis or a nasal allergy.

"*When do you get your colds?*"
If perennially in the spring or from the middle of August till frost, chances are good he is allergic to pollen. If in the late fall, there's a good possibility he is allergic to house dust — an even better possibility if the nasal obstruction and discharge begins in the fall and lasts *all* winter. If the patient is a child who gets a runny, stopped-up nose only when he is in school, he may be allergic to chalk dust (or maybe just "allergic" to school!).

Of course, sometimes the answers don't come too readily. Some people are sensitive to allergens they come in contact with only occasionally, so their reactions are more difficult to differentiate from colds. They may come from a new hair dye, or from fresh plaster and paint in a new house, or from a new fabric.

Do the cold-like symptoms occur only after eating eggs or after drinking a lot of milk? If so, I suspect allergy to protein, a common allergic offender.

"*Do any of your relatives have allergies?*"
Here, obviously, I'm looking for persistent headache, eczema, hives, cyclic vomiting, diarrhea, asthma, chronic cough, or nasal polyps. Psychic factors also seem to play a part in allergic reactions. Whereas colds affect all kinds of people in all walks of life, allergic upsets seem to occur most often in high-strung, intelligent people. Allergic nasal obstruction is sometimes a complication of menstruation, either as a result of physiologic changes or accompanying psychic stresses.

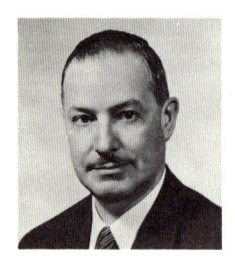

Raymond S. Rosedale, M.D.
Canton, Ohio

Doctor Rosedale is a member of the Senior Staff, Otolaryngology, and Chief of the Department of Plastic Surgery of the Head and Neck, Mercy Hospital and Timken-Mercy Hospital, in Canton, Ohio. He is a Diplomate of both the American Board of Pathology and the American Board of Otolaryngology. Included among his professional affiliations are the American Academy of Ophthalmology and Otolaryngology, and the American College of Allergists.

Clues from Examining the Nasal Mucosa

Both colds and nasal allergic reactions often begin with sneezing and a stopped-up nose. The nasal obstruction in a cold usually remains unilateral for 24 to 36 hours before the other side becomes involved, whereas in an allergic reaction the obstruction shifts frequently from side to side.

If the mucosa is violaceous-gray, boggy, and bathed in mucus, the disorder is almost always due to allergy. However, an allergy cannot be ruled out if the mucosa is *not* violaceous-gray and boggy. Sometimes the nasal mucosa of an allergic patient is brick-red and not especially swollen.

The discharge is usually watery in allergy, but sometimes globs of mucus may be seen in the midportion of the nasal chambers or in the posterior choanae. When a patient has a cold, his nasal mucosa is apt to be pomegranate-red and more distended. If the mucosa shrinks readily when sprayed with a weak cocaine solution, the disorder is more likely an allergy than a cold.

When the nasal disorder is allergic, his temperature will probably remain normal or only slightly elevated. He is much more likely to have a fever and suffer malaise with a cold.

Sure Means of Differentiation

Nasal polyps are a certain sign of nasal allergy. They are gray and glistening, and often multiple. They most often arise from the middle meatus. Vasoconstrictors will shrink nasal polyps, unless they have undergone fibrous dysplasia. Nasal polyps are characteristic findings in some cases of fibrocystic disease. Therefore, in children and adolescents this possibility may be investigated by determining the sodium and chloride content of the sweat.

Cytologic studies provide a sure differentiation if the history, symptoms, and signs leave you still in doubt. The presence of eosinophiles in mucus nets indicates allergy. With colds these are replaced by lymphocytes and, later, with secondary infection, by an increasing number of polymorphonuclear leukocytes.

Even when the patient does have a viral or bacterial infection, he may also have an allergic condition, so it is a good idea to treat the cold and then check again to see whether there are allergic manifestations after the infection has cleared. In either case, antihistamines and decongestants will not only make the patient more comfortable, but will also help differentiate; if the symptoms disappear or are markedly alleviated in a few hours or a day, the patient has probably had an allergic reaction, not a cold.

POSTNASAL DRIP

The dripping in postnasal drip usually results from a change in the viscosity of nasal and paranasal secretions. Usually they become slightly thinner, but not watery, and increase in volume. Drops form as the cilia lining the nasopharynx propel the secretions over the soft palate and down the uvula toward the esophagus. Sometimes the secretions become thicker, due to drying of the mucosa or low-grade infection, and are not carried off normally, forming droplets.

Intranasal Obstructions

Intranasal obstructions can also cause postnasal drip, so the nasal cavity should be examined carefully for such abnormal conditions as septal spurs and polyps, as well as occlusive deviations of the septum. If there are no obstructions, a change in viscosity is probably responsible for the condition, and successful treatment depends on finding its cause and correcting it.

Allergic Causes

Mild allergy or tissue sensitivity is a very common cause of postnasal drip. Unlike a severe allergy, where nasal discharge is persistent and profuse and suggests a "common cold," just enough secretion results to make the patient miserable.

Some means of telling an allergy from an infection are: the pale, grayish edematous appearance of the nasal mucous membrane; the watery discharge containing eosinophiles; a positive skin reaction; and improvement when the suspected agents are avoided. These signs are not present in nasal infections, unless the infection is secondary to an already-existing allergic process.

Postnasal drip may also be caused by local irritation without allergic involvement, such as inhaling tobacco smoke and other fumes. These irritants, disturbing enough to persons with a normal nasal mucosa, are especially disturbing to those with allergies.

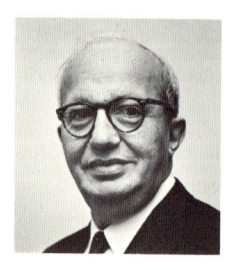

Albert P. Seltzer, M.D.
University of Pennsylvania

Doctor Seltzer is Associate Professor of Otolaryngology at the University of Pennsylvania Graduate School of Medicine; Chief of the Ear, Nose, and Throat Department at Mercy-Douglass Hospital; and Senior Attending Physician at Albert Einstein Medical Center in Philadelphia. He is a Fellow of the American College of Surgeons.

Low Humidity Dries Mucosa

Overheating and poor ventilation in the winter, with a resultant low humidity, lead to drying of the nasal mucosa. Secretions become more viscous, interfere with the activity of the cilia, and are not carried off normally. Droplets form and fall into the back of the throat. Mouth-breathing will sometimes have a similar effect, even when the inhaled air is not abnormally dry.

I have noticed that many people, especially older people, fall into the habit of drawing the secretions into the nasopharynx instead of blowing their noses. Then they try to clear the nasopharynx of this self-caused postnasal drip by noisily clearing their throats. Sometimes a postnasal drip can be cleared by so simple a measure as telling the patient to blow his nose more often.

Emotions can often be involved indirectly in postnasal drip. Depression, for example, is often accompanied by postnasal drip resulting from nasal and lacrimal secretions, which are partly controlled by sympathetic fibers from the cervical ganglion and from the trigeminal nerve.

Abnormal general physical conditions, such as disturbed elimination or endocrine imbalance, are less likely to cause postnasal drip but may be involved and must be suspected when other causes are not found.

High Pillow Helps

Overuse or unnecessary use of medicinal sprays can also cause postnasal drip. Their use often forces secretions backward into the nasopharynx. Stopping them and having the patient sleep on a high, rather than a flat, pillow should help considerably. I have checked the effect of different pillow heights on postnasal drip by instilling methylene blue in the anterior nasal chamber of patients at night. When they slept on high pillows, no methylene blue appeared in the expectorate the next morning, whereas it did when they slept on flat pillows.

Be certain to reassure your patient that postnasal drip, though unpleasant, is harmless. This reassurance may help eliminate the emotional aggravation that often is present. I have seen patients so aware of an irritation that caused them to clear their throats or cough frequently, that they were afraid they had cancer. Telling them they had a simple postnasal drip condition was like lifting the weight of the world from their shoulders. And, remember about the high pillow; it will help ease your patient's discomfort while you treat the cause of his postnasal drip.

"SINUS TROUBLE, DOCTOR"

When we ask a patient the usual question, "What's the trouble?" we often get the laconic reply, "Sinus, Doctor." Sometimes he amplifies his terse self-diagnosis to "Sinus trouble," and then we enter into a tug-of-war to pry out of him just what he means by this.

To the patient, "sinus trouble" may mean nasal discharge, nasal obstruction, pain in one or more areas of his face, or headache — or perhaps all of these. Before we can appraise his symptoms accurately, we have to untangle them and decide which ones constitute bona fide "sinus trouble" and which ones do not.

In order to understand "sinus trouble," we have to keep in mind the basic physiology and anatomy of the sinuses: they are air-containing cavities that develop as extensions of the nasal passages; they are lined with the same ciliated mucous membrane as the nose itself. Barring such rare conditions as osteomatous or malignant growths, almost all sinus disorders are due to changes in the structure of the lining membrane. This membrane is paper-thin and produces a mucous secretion; for it to function properly, it must be ventilated and able to drain by way of the natural ostia into the nasal cavities. As long as these openings are not obstructed by mucosal edema or inflammation, all is well; but any changes that block off the sinus cavities tend to produce symptoms that can truly be called "sinus trouble."

Frontal Sinusitis and "Headache"

Sinusitis is usually secondary to an acute upper respiratory infection. This is especially true of infection of the frontal sinuses. The tortuous passageway through which they usually drain is temporarily blocked by the swollen mucous membrane, and then absorption of air in the sinus creates a vacuum or negative pressure. This causes severe pain over one or both eyes. Strictly speaking, this is more accurately a pain over the eye rather than a headache, but the patient will usually complain of "headache." The pain of frontal sinusitis has a very characteristic and peculiar timing: it is absent on waking in the morning and develops,

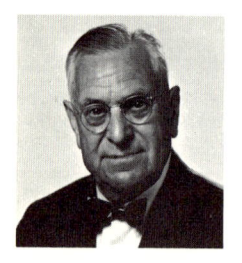

Lyman G. Richards, M.D.
Wellesley Hills, Massachusetts

Doctor Richards is Secretary of the American Laryngological Association. He received his medical education at Harvard Medical School, at St. Luke's Hospital, New York, and at the Massachusetts Eye and Ear Infirmary, Boston. He is a past president of the American Laryngological, Rhinological and Otological Society and also of the American Broncho-Esophagological Association.

often with clocklike precision, in the midmorning. Then it eases up or even disappears toward evening. The pain is often worse when the patient bends over or shakes his head, and there is acute tenderness to pressure over the upper, inner wall of the orbit.

Frontal sinusitis attacks are usually self-limited, lasting a week or 10 days. Any of the medications available to shrink the nasal mucous membranes will help, especially when supplemented with heat applied externally. If pain is severe, the patient may need sedation, though analgesics will usually suffice. There is seldom any marked fever, and antibiotics are usually not indicated.

The maxillary sinuses are affected and treated similarly. When obstruction causes maxillary sinusitis, there is pain over the cheek and along the alveolar ridge, radiating into the upper teeth. There is less pain than in frontal sinusitis, but until maxillary sinusitis subsides (in a week to 10 days) it may cause considerable discomfort when the patient chews.

Symptoms of ethmoiditis are less clear-cut and less localized than those of frontal or maxillary sinusitis, but generally there is a sense of congestion and fullness on one or both sides of the upper nasal cavities. Ethmoiditis usually is not painful. The sphenoidal sinuses, deep in the back of the nasal passages, are seldom involved in sinusitis. But when they are, the patient may complain of a deep-seated headache referred to the occipital region. Sphenoidal sinusitis is difficult to differentiate from other causes of headache in this area.

Sinusitis is usually short-lived and self-limited, subsiding shortly after the patient's head cold subsides. The discomfort and disability, if any, are brief. But when there is persistent obstruction to drainage and ventilation because of tissue changes, there may be a pathological change in the lining membrane of the involved sinuses; the lining may become thicker and there may be an accumulation of purulent yellowish exudate. Without treatment, the condition may become chronic, with marked hypertrophy of the sinus lining. Often the entire lumen is obliterated by the lining, which may form polypoid excrescences so large as to protrude through the sinus ostium into the nasal passages. Polyp formation is common in patients with an underlying allergy. Treatment, aside from removing the polyps — a surgical procedure that should be left to a rhinologist — requires control of the allergy.

Diagnosis

How, then, can we separate the patient's complaints of "sinus trouble" from those arising from conditions totally unrelated to the sinuses? First, we can inspect the nasal passages with a head mirror and reflected light. It takes patience and practice to develop skill with the head mirror, but once this is developed, this method of examination is far superior to the method of visualization afforded by any of the various electrical speculae. With reflected light from the head mirror, you can see whether the airway is adequate, whether there is any obstruction of the sinuses by high unilateral deviation of the septum, whether the middle turbinate impinges on the middle meatus (common area of drainage for the antrum, ethmoids, and frontal sinuses), whether there is purulent discharge, and whether there is any polyposis or actual polyp formation. Only a rhinologist is likely to be able to evaluate minor changes in nasal structure, but any physician can detect clearly pathological conditions.

Second, transillumination should be done in a completely darkened room, using one of the transilluminating lights designed for the purpose. You should hold the bulb just inside the lower rim of the orbit and consider the translucency viewed through the homolateral hard palate. If there is opacity or little translucency, the diminution is usually due to thickened lining membrane or purulent fluid in the maxillary antra. Rarely, you may see *increased* translucency, caused by a cyst containing clear fluid.

Transillumination is less useful in studying the frontal sinuses because they are seldom as symmetrical as the maxillary sinuses, and because they vary in size and shape. When they are translucent, there is no pathological condition, but when they are not, it may be due to the small size or even absence of the sinus. Transillumination does not help in studying the ethmoidal and sphenoid sinuses.

Third, X-rays can provide accurate information about all the sinuses, but for best results they should be taken and interpreted by a specialist. To hold down the patient's medical expenses, you may prefer to use X-ray only as a last resort, but X-rays should never be omitted when the diagnosis is in doubt.

Complications

Conservative measures that re-establish normal ventilation and drainage will clear up most sinusitis due to uncomplicated infection of the nasal passages. Sometimes, however, pain and tenderness disappear but nasal discharge, usually purulent, persists. When this happens, and transillumination shows that the maxillary antrum is opaque from accumulated fluid, you may have to irrigate the sinus with a saline solution to which an antibiotic powder has been added. Many physicians will prefer to have this done by a rhinologist, depending on their familiarity with irrigation procedures, especially when it is impossible to insert a cannula into the natural ostium. When the cannula cannot be inserted, the only way to irrigate the sinus is to introduce a needle through the thin bony wall of the inferior meatus. After one or more irrigations by either method, the return fluid will no longer be purulent, but will be a clear, straw-colored liquid with a consistency like the yolk of an egg. This is an almost certain indication that the lining membrane has returned to normal.

The frontal sinus and — though it is less accessible — the sphenoid can be irrigated similarly, though the location of their ostia makes it more difficult to irrigate them than the maxillary. Fortunately, they are less likely to accumulate purulent fluid.

Chronic hypertrophy and polyp formation involving the sinus lining present far more difficult problems and may require surgery. They call for the opinion of a specialist.

In my experience, only a small percentage of patients complaining of "sinus trouble" actually have any true sinus abnormality. The physician in general practice, viewing the whole patient, is in as good a position as a specialist to separate sinus disease from the host of other causes of headache or nasal discharge. The rhinologist, despite his best intentions, sometimes finds it difficult not to view the entire patient through the all-too-narrow aperture of his head mirror. Once you have determined that there is a pathological intranasal condition, though, his help may be needed and it surely will if it becomes necessary to do surgery or a sinus puncture.

chapter 3

COMPLAINTS ABOUT THE STOMACH

OBSCURE ABDOMINAL PAIN

This is more a check-list than an article. You might think of it as a catalogue of clues to the riddle of the "Great Abdominal Mimics," a list of non-gastrointestinal disorders that are apt to lie behind the confusing clinical, laboratory, and radiographic features of acute and chronic abdominal pain. Over the years, this check-list approach has frequently helped me to avoid serious diagnostic error and fruitless surgery.

Nine Things to Remember

In the first place, there are nine things that I tell myself to do whenever I see a patient in consultation for obscure abdominal pain.

1. Seek out significant familial disease in close relatives.

2. Carefully check the skin and mucous membranes for possible clues to a systemic disorder.

3. Pay attention to the ancillary X-ray findings.

4. When pertinent, pursue the psychodynamic approach, including an interview with a key member of the patient's family.

5. Keep in mind possible relationships among seemingly unrelated disorders (such as peptic ulcer with functional hyperinsulinism or hyperparathyroidism, and thyroiditis or the Sjögren syndrome with connective-tissue disorders).

6. Repeatedly review the accumulated data on patients followed for prolonged periods.

7. Repeat the *complete* physical examination at reasonable intervals.

8. Keep in mind the possibility of a new and unrelated complicating disorder when there is an unexplained change in patients with adequately controlled chronic diseases (e.g., diabetes, pernicious anemia).

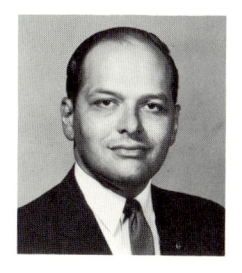

Hyman J. Roberts, M.D.
West Palm Beach, Florida

Doctor Roberts is a former Research Fellow and Instructor in Medicine at the Tufts University and Georgetown Medical Schools. He currently is on the Consulting Staff of Good Samaritan Hospital and St. Mary's Hospital in West Palm Beach, Florida. He is a Diplomate of the American Board of Internal Medicine, a Fellow of the American College of Chest Physicians, and an Associate of the American College of Physicians.

9. Question the results of equivocal or inappropriate results of laboratory tests, and do not hesitate to repeat the test.

Using these nine basic points as a framework of reference, I consider the following "check-list" of the more important systemic causes of obscure abdominal pain.

Endocrinopathies

√ *Adrenal* — Consider the possibility of primary, symptomatic, or iatrogenic *adrenocortical insufficiency* in the patient with unexplained abdominal or costovertebral pain, whether or not he has nausea, vomiting, or pigmentation of the skin or mucous membranes. If he is receiving an adrenocortical steroid, his abdominal pain may be caused by peptic ulcer (a new ulcer or a reactivated one), pancreatitis, or collapse of osteoporotic vertebrae.

If the patient is diabetic, polycythemic or hypertensive, suspect that peptic ulcer may be symptomatic of *adrenocortical hyperfunction*. In young diabetic or hypertensive patients, also consider the possibility of *pheochromocytoma*. The high concentrations of norepinephrine produced by this tumor can cause necrotizing arteritis in the gastrointestinal wall, leading to hemorrhage or perforation.

√ *Thyroid* — Remember the possibility of *hypothyroidism*, especially in patients who have had a thyroidectomy or radioactive iodine. I am amazed at how often and for how long this readily treatable condition is overlooked under these circumstances. Atypical *hyperthyroidism* can also manifest itself as abdominal pain, diarrhea, and vague abdominal symptoms — particularly in elderly persons with an "apathetic" demeanor.

√ *Parathyroid* — Unexplained epigastric burning or pain, recurrent and refractory peptic ulceration, and pancreatitis are common in patients with *hyperparathyroidism*. A refractory or recurrent duodenal ulcer in a female poses an important clue to hyperparathyroidism. Remember that the results of calcium and phosphorus determinations, even when repeated, can be misleading unless the laboratory is expert in performing them.

√ *Pancreas* — Consider an ulcerogenic tumor of the pancreas (Zollinger-Ellison syndrome) in any patient with multiple ulcers of the stomach, duodenum, or jejunum which recur in spite of surgery and careful medical management. Such a tumor may or may not cause associated diarrhea.

Metabolic Disorders

√ *Metabolic disorders* that commonly cause severe abdominal pain or other gastrointestinal symptoms include: chronic renal disease, hemochromatosis, porphyria, hypercalcemia, hyperlipemia, familial recurring Mediterranean fever, functional hyperinsulinism, and diabetes mellitus. I should like to emphasize the importance of *functional ("diabetogenic") hyperinsulinism* as a major etiology in the genesis of duodenal ulcer (especially among women) and "psychophysiologic gastrointestinal phenomena," and as a frequently treatable aggravating factor in "refractory" chronic ulcerative colitis and regional enteritis.

Toxic Reactions

√ *Lead poisoning* — Deserves serious consideration in communities with many old homes (painted with lead oxide paint) and among employees of lead-using industries (painters, printers, automobile body and storage battery workers). A new source of lead poisoning, recently prevalent in the southeastern United States, is the ingestion of illegal whiskey that has been processed through car radiators.

√ *Arsenic poisoning* — May cause abdominal pain and obscure melena. In such patients, abdominal X-rays will show the dense, radiopaque material.

√ *Drug reactions* — Consider especially the following: digitalis, aspirin, anticholinergics (particularly in unrecognized pyloroduodenal obstruction), chlorothiazide or hydrochlorothiazides containing postassium, adrenocortical steroids (see above), reserpine, hypoprothrombinemic anticoagulants (even without overt bleeding), phenylbutazone, drugs that cause urinary retention, and drugs that affect liver function (including extrahepatic cholestasis).

√ *Drug addiction* — A relatively uncommon cause of abdominal pain, but should receive special consideration in medical and paramedical personnel. A provocative test with nalorphine may confirm this suspicion.

Infections

√ *Bacterial endocarditis* — Consider S.B.E. in any patient with a significant heart murmur and fever. The abdominal pain may be due to a diaphragmatic pleuritis secondary to pulmonary embolism, or to mesenteric or splenic embolization. Persistent left-upper-quadrant pain and bacteremia after intensive antibiotic therapy may be due to infection within a splenic infarct.

√ *Tuberculosis* — Consider it seriously in susceptible ethnic groups, in patients with debilitating disease, in those previously treated for tuberculosis, in those receiving adrenocortical steroids, and in recently parturient women. Tuberculous mesenteric or retroperitoneal lymphadenitis also can cause abdominal pain. Remember that, occasionally, patients with active tuberculosis do not give a positive tuberculin reaction.

√ *Infectious mononucleosis* — Causes abdominal pain through hyperplasia of the abdominal lymph nodes, hepatomegaly or pancreatitis.

√ *Viral hepatitis* — Its long incubation period may add to the diagnostic difficulty. It sometimes helps to remember that hepatitis does not always cause clinical jaundice. In patients previously maintained uneventfully on long-term anticoagulant therapy, consider the possibility of unexplained bleeding as the first sign of a complicating hepatitis.

√ *Herpes zoster* — It is notoriously able to simulate abdominal emergencies in its pre-eruptive phase, even causing acute intestinal obstruction.

Hematologic and Cardiovascular Disorders

√ *Myeloma* — Always consider it in patients with unexplained abdominal pain and anemia, particularly in males over 40 with extensive osteoporosis. Myeloma causes pain by: nerve compression by a collapsed vertebra, extramedullary tumor formation, perineural invasion, spinal cord involvement, hypercalcemia (which may respond dramatically to corticosteroid), or complicating amyloidosis.

√ *Sickle-cell anemia* — It and its variants are the "great abdominal masqueraders" among Negroes. So *always* look for sickle-cell disease before you recommend surgery for any Negro patient in whom you suspect a perforated peptic ulcer, intestinal obstruction, acute pancreatitis, or renal or biliary disease. At high altitudes, patients with sickle-cell hemoglobin C disease develop abdominal pain due to splenic infarction.

√ *Polycythemia vera* — May cause abdominal pain as a result of peptic ulcer, mesenteric thrombosis, hepatic congestion, or splenic infarction. Consider this diagnosis whenever severe hemorrhage from a peptic ulcer is followed by relatively normal hemograms before there has been enough time for the blood volume to adjust. However, do not attribute hematuria and abdominal pain solely to polycythemia vera until you have excluded symptomatic erythrocytosis secondary to a renal carcinoma.

It is especially important to consider polycythemia in pre-surgical patients. When polycythemic patients undergo abdominal surgery without previous venesection, their postoperative period may be complicated by mesenteric vascular occlusion (arterial or venous), thrombosis of the hepatic veins (possibly resulting in the Budd-Chiari syndrome), or extensive thrombosis of the portal vein.

√ *Coronary heart disease* — Can closely mimic an acute abdominal emergency. It is often overlooked until after unnecessary surgery. A preoperative electrocardiogram could establish this diagnosis; unfortunately, the EKG is often omitted because pericarditis commonly occurs in young adults in whom we do not usually expect heart disease.

√ *Abdominal angina (intermittent mesenteric ischemia)* — Typically causes epigastric pain that occurs within one-half to one hour after eating. The pain may radiate to the subcostal and lumbar areas; it is relieved by lying on the side, or by leaning forward in the sitting position (which reduces the drag on the mesentery). Mesenteric ischemia may be due to an embolus, portal hypertension, polyarteritis, peripheral vascular collapse, congestive heart failure, cardiac arrhythmias, and either myocardial infarction or its treatment (pressor agents).

√ *Pulmonary embolism* — Causes upper abdominal pain that simulates gallbladder colic, subdiaphragmatic abscess, hepatitis, and other abdominal emergencies. The diagnosis is especially difficult when the onset of pleuritic pain or hemoptysis is delayed.

√ *Dissecting aneurysm of the aorta* — Often causes symptoms that initially suggest peptic ulcer, acute pancreatitis, acute cholecystitis, mesenteric thrombosis, or even abdominal tumors. Although dissection usually occurs in older patients with hypertension, it may also occur in relatively young persons (notably in association with pregnancy or polycystic disease of the kidneys and liver). It occasionally goes unrecognized for a long time.

Connective Tissue Diseases

√ *Systemic lupus erythematosus* — May be suspected first by the pathologist who studies tissue removed at laparotomy that was performed for persistent or acute abdominal pain. S.L.E. can cause intestinal ulceration, mesenteric artery thrombosis, disorders of the liver and its capsule, lesions of the spleen, pancreatitis, or retroperitoneal bleeding. Consider this possibility especially in young women with joint or lung symptoms, fever, a false-positive serologic test for syphilis, hypergammaglobulinemia, or a suggestive family history (notably on the maternal side). In this clinical setting, a pathology report of "hyperplastic lymphadenopathy" is a significant clue to systemic lupus.

√ *Polyarteritis (periarteritis nodosa)* also may be first suspected by the pathologist — usually in his report on a removed appendix or gallbladder. In patients with polyarteritis, a hemorrhagic infarct in the jejunum or ileum may cause ulceration or perforation of the bowel. Infarction of the pancreas may cause abdominal pain radiating to the back.

Nervous System Disorders

√ *"Functional disorders"* — A source of all kinds of gastrointestinal distress, so remember to look for signs of neurosis in patients whose symptoms seem to have no physical cause. However, *avoid* classifying recent complaints in individuals over 40 as "psychophysiologic" until after thorough study and an adequate follow-up period. *Carcinoma of the cecum, the right colon and the pancreas can behave notoriously like functional disease in their early stages.* Similarly, *reactive hypoglycemia is a commonly overlooked, readily definable, and easily treated* "physiologic" component in such patients.

√ *"Ambulatory schizophrenia"* — Often the basis of recurrent abdominal distress and bizarre visceral complaints. Consider it in patients who describe their symptoms vaguely, who bring in a stack of negative laboratory examinations, who are extremely self-conscious, and who have long-impaired social adaptation. Similarly, consider "pseudo-allergic schizophrenia" in patients who attribute chronically recurrent abdominal pain to food allergy; such patients usually have a history of striking remission with various (and contradictory) diets and drugs.

√ *"Abdominal migraine"* (recurrent abdominal pain with associated nausea) — Can occur without an accompanying headache; it is common in postmenopausal women. So consider this cause in patients with the compulsive, driving, "migrainous personality." Consider it in children whose *parents* have migraine, and you will often spare them needless diagnostic studies. Suspect associated recurrent hypoglycemia due to functional hyperinsulinism or early diabetes mellitus if the disorder is nocturnal or if there is also a peptic ulcer.

√ *"Small strokes"* — Frequently cause obscure abdominal pain associated with other vague symptoms (e.g., burning of the tongue, a bad taste, the loss of interest, sleep disturbances, a general "slowing-up," and changes in memory). So always keep this possibility in mind when treating elderly patients.

THAT SO-CALLED INTRACTABLE ULCER

Most patients with peptic ulcer disease referred to me have failed to respond to treatment. What treatment failed? Usually I find it was something like the following:
- three bland meals a day
- a snack or glass of milk between meals
- antacid tablets before and after meals
- antispasmodics or anticholinergics and sedatives

This regimen is hazardous because it is just effective enough to encourage its routine use. On the average, 4 out of 5 patients will do well on it. But the remaining patient simply gets worse: his pain returns; his ulcer enlarges or penetrates. Eventually he may require surgery — surgery that with better treatment might have been avoided, or at least postponed long enough to permit a safe and definitive procedure to be performed.

In contrast, almost all patients will respond if a "stomach rest" regimen is followed. I recently had the occasion to review the case histories of 100 outpatients who had been referred for treatment of their ulcer. For weeks, months, or even years in some, they had been on a regimen similar to that outlined above. (One man with a penetrating ulcer had been hospitalized for six months in a psychiatric ward for "functional back pain.") But in all of them, in spite of the duration of their illness, a "stomach rest" regimen relieved daytime symptoms, usually by the end of 12 to 48 hours. For those who had symptoms continuously for several months or even longer, it required four to six days. In the management of early uncomplicated peptic ulcer, one can expect "stomach rest" to relieve symptoms much more rapidly; about 12 hours is the rule.

The Principle of "Stomach Rest"

The principle of rest is one of the common denominators in all medical treatment. When the heart has been damaged by a coronary occlusion, we cannot stop it from contracting, but we can limit the burden imposed

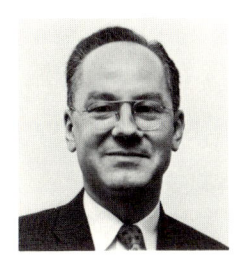

James L. A. Roth, M.D., Ph.D.
University of Pennsylvania

Doctor Roth is Professor of Clinical Gastroenterology and Director of the Division of Gastroenterology at the Graduate School of Medicine and Graduate Hospital, University of Pennsylvania. He is a director of gastrointestinal research and Chief of the Gastrointestinal Clinic at the Graduate Hospital. His professional affiliations include the American Gastroenterological Association and the American College of Physicians.

upon it by restricting the activity of the patient. The same can be done with the ulcerated stomach or duodenum.

To promote healing, especially in the early stages, the stomach should be kept in a state of relative rest. The regimen used to accomplish this state of rest is based on the classic studies of A. J. Carlson, who found the introduction of a feeding temporarily inhibits peristaltic activity. This phenomenon he called receptive relaxation. The most vigorous peristaltic contractions, of course, occur in the empty stomach (hunger), and the next most vigorous are encountered as the stomach attempts to empty its contents after a full meal. Hourly small feedings, however, will avoid these extremes of motor activity and will repeatedly bring about receptive relaxation, thus maintaining a state of relative "stomach rest." In the early management of active peptic ulcer, the objective of treatment should be to keep the stomach and duodenum in this state.

The Regimen

For most ambulatory patients, the regimen is begun with the ever-available milk feeding, 5 ounces every hour on the hour during the waking hours. When convenient, a similar quantity of Cream of Wheat®, creamed soup of vegetable puree, Jello®, custard or pudding may be substituted for the milk. On the half hour, midway between feedings, peristalsis begins to return only to be inhibited again by the ingestion of liquid or powdered antacids. Initially, I prefer liquid antacids to the tablets, because they mix more readily with gastric content and are more efficient in their capacity to neutralize the hydrochloric acid. Needless to say, the use of tobacco, alcohol and caffeine beverages is forbidden.

During this phase of management, I give a mild sedative, and to further reduce motor activity, a tolerance dose of an anticholinergic. By a tolerance dose, I mean *all* the anticholinergic the patient can tolerate without experiencing undue side effects. There is no "standard dose" of an anticholinergic agent. The amount prescribed should be determined by titrating the dose for each patient individually. The dose should be maintained just below that level which will cause blurring of vision. Such a "stomach rest" regimen is employed for 10 to 14 days before permitting any additional food items. Then gradually over a period of two months or so, the diet is advanced with stepwise increments providing five small meals and eventually three meals of bland, low-residue food with milk feedings between meals.

The Regimen Not Inconvenient

I have treated doctors, lawyers, mechanics, taxicab drivers — all have carried their thermos of milk around with them in the initial phase of their management, and they are glad to do it. After all, they have spent a great deal of time and money without getting any results, and are only too happy to follow a regimen that works. So with patient cooperation presenting no problem, the majority of them can remain ambulatory. However, if they do not respond in a week's time, I hospitalize them. Getting them away from their home environment, business or other emotional strain is sometimes necessary before they respond to treatment.

Of course, when there is a confined perforation, the ulcer may heal temporarily only to break down as the diet is advanced in the second or third month. Surgery is frequently required in this group of patients. A period of preoperative "stomach rest" will usually permit the edema and inflammation to subside so that the surgery itself will be easier technically. Thus, the surgeon can perform a definitive procedure, such as a hemigastrectomy with vagotomy or a three-quarter gastric resection. Otherwise, in the presence of a massive inflammatory reaction about a confined perforation, he may be forced to do a pyloric exclusion, or a gastroenterostomy and vagotomy. These compromise procedures are followed by a higher incidence of recurrent ulceration or gastric stasis.

Stomach Acid: How Important?

The dictum "no acid, no active peptic ulcer" has never been refuted, and there is no doubt that acid is essential to the pathogenesis of peptic ulceration. However, the level of free acid in the stomach remains relatively constant whether the ulcer is active or in remission. Thus, it would appear that a breakdown in mucosal resistance is an even more important factor in ulcer genesis. Furthermore, the relative importance of acid is revealed by the observation that even a "stomach rest" regimen, while it affords as effective a control of acid as possible, usually suppresses acid only slightly. I think we have deluded ourselves into thinking hourly feedings, hourly antacids, and tolerance doses of anticholinergic can be depended upon to eliminate the acid factor. On the other hand, in spite of the relatively high level of acidity, the "stomach rest" regimen does facilitate ulcer healing. Many of the measures used to suppress secretion also depress motor activity. So, it would appear that avoiding mucosal irritants and putting the stomach and duodenum at motor rest are of greater importance in promoting ulcer healing than our ineffective, though desirable, efforts which only partially neutralize the acid.

chapter 4

COMPLAINTS ABOUT THE EYES

VAGUE COMPLAINTS ABOUT EYESIGHT

Many patients seen by general practitioners have vague complaints about their eyesight, such as "My vision seems cloudy at times," "I don't think I can see as well as I used to," and "Sometimes things look crooked . . . I don't know whether it's my imagination or not."

Can you tell how serious these and similar common complaints are, and what they mean? Should such patients be referred to an ophthalmologist? Are there some criteria to help decide which ones do not need to be referred?

In this article, I would like to answer some of these questions, to help you deal with common complaints about eyesight.

"I have trouble seeing at night . . ."

Severe night blindness is usually caused by retinitis pigmentosa and always deserves investigation. The other possible cause, vitamin A deficiency, is easily remedied by adequate intake of the vitamin. Retinitis pigmentosa is congenital, but usually does not progress far enough to be recognized until the patient is an adult. The *first* symptom is night blindness, which increases in severity. Characteristically, when you examine the patient's eye, you will find that the retinal vessels are markedly attenuated, that the optic nerve has atrophied and looks dirty gray, and that the disk appears pale and waxy. You will usually find pigmentary changes — spots of color — of varying extent in the mid-periphery of the fundus which are described as bone corpuscle pigmentation because of their spidery appearance. As the disease progresses, cataracts develop and the visual field constricts until only a small central island of vision remains.

I know of no effective treatment for retinitis pigmentosa. Dr. Dan M. Gordon, of Cornell University Medical College, says he uses vasodilators to counteract the attenuation of retinal vessels. Sometimes the patient can be helped by removing the cataract when one forms, but this can be considered a delaying action only, for the typical patient's vision will continue to deteriorate.

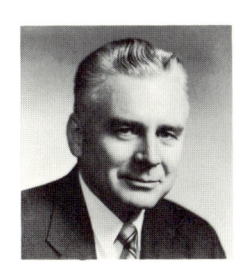

Harold G. Scheie, M.D.
University of Pennsylvania

Doctor Scheie is Professor of Ophthalmology at the University of Pennsylvania School of Medicine, and he has served on the National Medical Foundation for Eye Care. His professional affiliations include the American Academy of Ophthalmology and Otolaryngology, the American Ophthalmological Society, the Association for Research in Ophthalmology, and the Board of Regents of the American College of Surgeons.

"My eyes water all the time..."

When a patient, young or old, complains of excessive lacrimation, but no other symptoms, it is probably due to obstructed drainage through the nasolacrimal apparatus rather than to overproduction of tears. An adult with this condition may need surgery: anastomosis of the lacrimal sac with the nose to provide a new drainage channel. An infant with this condition usually needs only to have the tear duct probed; the obstruction usually results from failure of the nasolacrimal duct to open beneath the inferior turbinate.

An infant's tear ducts should not be probed until he is about five months old, however, even though excessive tearing from obstruction may be accompanied by mucopurulent secretion on the lid margins and lashes. I say this because in many cases the duct will open spontaneously by the time the child is five or six months old. Before that age, the condition should be managed conservatively by bathing the eye with physiologic saline solution.

When excessive lacrimation is accompanied by redness of the eye, it is probably due to irritation from conjunctivitis, a foreign body, or corneal ulceration. There is usually pain, photophobia, and blurring of vision, too. In children under one year, this combination of lacrimation and redness of the eye may be due to infantile glaucoma, so you should rule this out before you consider any other cause.

"My child's eyes seem crooked..."

If a child is more than six months of age and one eye deviates from the visual axis, the cause is probably a nonparalytic strabismus associated with an error of refraction. A child's strabismus can, however, be associated with intracranial disease or injury that has paralyzed ocular muscles. Therefore, any child with strabismus should be referred promptly to an ophthalmologist. A cause of strabismus is retinoblastoma, a common tumor of the eye, which can invade the macula. Early diagnosis here can be lifesaving. In adults, when one eye deviates from the optical axis, diplopia usually occurs and usually means that the patient has some organic neurological disease.

"I often have pain behind my eyes..."

Recurring headaches can be due to many things, including something wrong with the patient's eyes. Consider refractive error, vertical muscle imbalance, and glaucoma. Even if headache is not due to any of these, the eye often provides the clue to other diseases, especially those of neurological origin — revealed by papilledema and visual-field deficiencies — or vascular origin — revealed by eyeground examination. It is a good idea to ask the patient if his headache is localized behind one or both eyes. If it is, ask him if the pain gets worse when he rotates his eyes. If it does, very likely the cause is retrobulbar or optic neuritis.

"I sometimes see circles around lights..."

When a patient says he sees circles or colored halos around lights, chances are that he has either acute glaucoma or a cataract. It is possible, of course, that the halos may be produced by mucus on the cornea, edema from corneal dystrophy, but the fact that glaucoma *may* be the cause makes it imperative that it be considered first, for glaucoma should be treated early. The halos, from any cause, look to the patient somewhat like those we all see around street lights in foggy weather. In glaucoma, the halo effect comes from edema in the corneal epithelium caused by the rapid rise of intraocular pressure. In nuclear cataracts, the halo effect is caused by pigment deposits in the lens.

"My vision seems cloudy..." "I see spots..." "I'm losing my eyesight..."

A panorama of eye diseases can disturb vision, but a few specific complaints suggest specific diagnoses and these are worth keeping in mind. One thing to ask the patient is whether visual loss was sudden or gradual. Another thing to ask is whether it comes and goes. Inflammation, circulatory change, and trauma all produce sudden visual loss. When inflammation is the cause, other signs and symptoms — redness and pain, for example — are usually prominent. When trauma produces visual loss, cause and effect are even more obvious.

There are other conditions, however — occlusion of a retinal vessel, vitreous or macular hemorrhage, or retinal detachment — that are more difficult to diagnose. Retinal detachment is also associated with a cloud or curtain over part of the visual field, with various degrees of visual-field loss. The patient may notice that his vision is better in the morning, and he may report that he sees flashes of light or that he suddenly notices spots before his eyes. Any patient who complains of seeing flashes of light *and* suddenly seeing spots before his eyes may have a retinal detachment or a retinal tear that can lead to detachment. Uveitis also causes spots before the eyes, however, and sometimes we can find nothing to account for the spots patients say they see.

The two commonest causes of gradual, progressive loss of vision, especially in older patients, are cataracts and macular degeneration. Cataracts can easily be removed surgically. Senile macular degeneration cannot be treated, but it does not lead to total blindness.

"Things looked curved..."

If a patient complains that he sees curved lines where he knows they should be straight — the edge of a doorway, for example — or of seeing a larger image with one eye than with the other, he has some kind of pathological condition of the retina (probably in the macular region).

The Most Important Point to Remember

I want to emphasize one extremely important point: remember to look for symptoms of glaucoma in all of your patients with visual disturbances, no matter what they are. This disease is one of the most common causes of blindness. I have already mentioned colored halos seen around lights by people with glaucoma. Other important symptoms of acute glaucoma are severe pain, redness of the eye, and a semidilated pupil. Nausea and vomiting are also common symptoms, and unfortunately these often mask the ocular symptoms to the extent that the patient may be treated for days or even a week or two for "gastrointestinal disease." A delay in specific treatment can be costly, for if an acute attack is neglected, blindness usually results. Therefore, if you are called upon to treat a patient whose predominant symptoms are nausea and vomiting, be sure to check for accompanying ocular symptoms. If they are present, intraocular pressure can be controlled with miotic agents, carbonic anhydrase inhibitors, and hypertonic agents such as urea. Once the pressure is under control, the patient can be referred to an ophthalmologist for surgery.

By contrast with the dramatic symptoms of acute glaucoma, chronic simple glaucoma is almost symptomless. It is difficult for even a highly trained specialist to diagnose, and it cannot be diagnosed positively without repeated tonometry, continuing observation, and provocative tests.

Even though diagnosis is difficult, if you suspect a patient has chronic glaucoma, the diagnosis should be made before intraocular pressure progresses to the point that it causes cupping of the optic nerve. With cupping there is loss of vision, which cannot be restored even though further loss be prevented. If acute glaucoma is diagnosed early, it can be cured by simple, safe peripheral iridectomy, an operation free of late complications. The chronic type should be treated medically if it is possible to control the pressure by this means.

* * *

I hope that this discussion will help you in diagnosing eye disease in your practice. We all need to learn more about such diseases to prevent needless cases of blindness.

EYE INFLAMMATION

Eye inflammation is a serious problem; it can result in loss of vision or even loss of an eye if it is not diagnosed and managed correctly. Fortunately, although correct diagnosis can at times be difficult, it can usually be done by simple techniques; all that is needed is some fluorescein, a pen light, and a magnifying loupe. The main causes of eye inflammation are conjunctivitis, iritis, uveitis, acute glaucoma, and corneal involvement such as keratitis or a foreign body. In this article, I will outline some methods for differentiating among them and for treating the inflammation.

Conjunctivitis — The Most Common Cause

By far the most common cause of eye inflammation is acute conjunctivitis resulting from viral or bacterial infection. The patient may also have an upper respiratory infection, or just have had one, or you may learn in taking the history that someone in his family has had a "bad cold." His symptoms will usually be relatively trivial: he will complain of a burning sensation in his eye, or say that his eye feels "scratchy" or that he has something in it. Most patients with conjunctivitis find their eyelids stuck together in the morning by a mucopurulent discharge dried on the eyelashes. When preauricular adenopathy is present, the patient most likely has acute conjunctivitis, and it is probably of viral origin. There is little, if any, photophobia. There is no change in pupil size.

A patient with conjunctivitis should be treated for at least 24 hours with broad-range antibiotics in solution or with an ointment instilled every two hours. A number of useful topical antibiotics, alone or in combination, are available commercially. Those not used for systemic therapy are preferable, because they avoid the possibility of sensitizing the patient. Preparations containing penicillin especially should be avoided, because of penicillin's high allergenic potential.

Bacterial conjunctivitis usually improves dramatically in a day or two. If symptoms persist, and especially if they *increase* after 48 hours, you will want to get an opinion from an ophthalmologist. The great

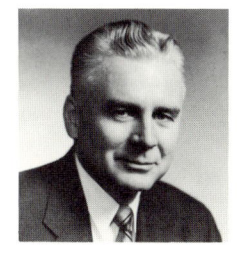

Harold G. Scheie, M.D.
University of Pennsylvania

Doctor Scheie is Professor of Ophthalmology at the University of Pennsylvania School of Medicine, and he has served on the National Medical Foundation for Eye Care. His professional affiliations include the American Academy of Ophthalmology and Otolaryngology, the American Ophthalmological Society, the Association for Research in Ophthalmology, and the Board of Regents of the American College of Surgeons.

danger in conjunctivitis is wrong diagnosis or associated corneal ulceration, which can complicate the infection and endanger vision.

Acute Glaucoma — Another Common Cause

Another common cause of eye inflammation is acute glaucoma. When symptoms are typical, diagnosis is easy, but when they are atypical or obscured by other signs, diagnosis can be difficult. The typical history includes recollections of previous mild prodromal attacks of blurring of vision and halos around lights, with or without ocular pain. These attacks have usually occurred under conditions that lead to pupillary dilatation — for example, while the patient was watching television in a dimly lighted room or movies in the darkness of a theater. Previous attacks may have disappeared spontaneously when the patient went into a lighted room or went to sleep.

The typical acute attack of glaucoma causes the patient to seek medical attention because of extreme pain and diminution of vision. The pain may be associated with marked nausea and vomiting; in fact, the gastrointestinal symptoms frequently predominate and obscure the ocular condition.

In addition to an inflamed eye, patients with acute glaucoma have semidilated pupils and the cornea is hazy with edema from high pressure. The pupils will react to neither light nor accommodation. The eye will feel very hard when palpated. Acute glaucoma is a medical emergency and an ophthalmologist should be called in promptly. You can, however, instill miotic agents as a first-aid measure. Once the intraocular pressure is normalized, these patients should undergo surgery.

Iritis and Anterior Uveitis — Produce Variable Symptoms

Iritis and anterior uveitis are other causes of eye inflammation that bring the patient to a physician. When typical, the inflamed area is circumcorneal or ciliary in type. The redness is most intense near the limbus and tends to fade away peripherally on the globe. Symptoms may vary remarkably, but usually the patient has severe deep ocular pain and photophobia. The pupil of his inflamed eye is almost always smaller than the other. His vision may or may not be blurred. Usually only one eye is affected, but occasionally both are. There is little ocular discharge, except for lacrimation. The lashes do not mat together. Such a patient should be referred to an ophthalmologist who will prescribe atropine and probably local or even systemic steroids. Atropine, and mydriatics in general, should be used very cautiously because of the very serious consequences if, by chance, the patient happens to have narrow-angle glaucoma.

Trauma — Easy to Diagnose

One of the more easily diagnosed causes of eye inflammation is trauma. This possible cause, of course, will be discovered in taking the history. Contusion of the eyeball can be followed by severe iritis, with the classic findings of that disease as described in the preceding section. You should question the patient carefully about the possibility of an intraocular foreign body, which can result in iritis or a frank purulent infection. If he has been hammering hard objects with a steel hammer, or if he has been working where there is any possibility of fragments being propelled through the air at high speed, the inflamed eye should be X-rayed.

After a contusion or penetrating injury of the globe, blood may be present (hyphemia) in the anterior chamber. This is a very serious sign. Secondary or recurring bleeding tends to occur, especially from the third to the seventh day after injury. This may result in severe secondary glaucoma with blood staining of the cornea and loss of vision or even of the eye. When there is hyphemia or evidence of any serious ocular trauma, you should request ophthalmologic consultation. Management is very exacting, placing heavy demands on specialized judgment.

Foreign Body and Keratitis — Two Corneal Conditions

Two common corneal conditions can result in a red, inflamed eye. The first and more common is a foreign body in the cornea, and the other is keratitis (inflammation of the cornea). An imbedded foreign body usually produces pain, but not always. If its presence is not obvious, a corneal foreign body can be detected by shining a pen light at the limbus or edge of the cornea and looking at the eye with a loupe. A light brought slowly to the limbus illuminates the foreign body, reflecting light rays to the examiner's eye that ordinarily are transmitted across the cornea to the opposite limbus by internal reflection. Any opacity in the cornea does the same thing, so the method is also excellent for detecting corneal infiltrates or ulcers.

When you cannot detect a foreign body in the cornea, it may be located beneath the tarsal plate of the upper lid and can be found easily by everting the lid with a cotton applicator. If nothing is found in either place, the cornea should be stained with fluorescein, which detects epithelial breaks, to exclude corneal abrasion or ulceration. Both corneal foreign bodies and keratitis, through the mechanism of axon reflexes, can cause histamine release and vasodilatation in the iris, with a reflex iritis and contraction of the pupil.

If you find a foreign body beneath the upper lid, you can easily wipe it away with a cotton applicator. A corneal foreign body can be much more difficult to manage and should be treated as a potential corneal ulcer. First, it should be removed with a moist applicator. Then the patient should be instructed to use antibiotic drops every two or three hours for two or three days or until the epithelial site heals. If rust-ring or staining remains after the foreign body is wiped away, this must be removed by an ophthalmologist. If you cannot dislodge the foreign body with an applicator, you will have to use a sharp instrument or a spud. In difficult cases, referral is advisable. The ophthalmologist will remove it with a sharp instrument such as a knife needle or the tip of a scalpel, and will employ a slit-lamp microscope for magnification in order to work with the least possible chance of injuring the cornea.

General Principles

Here are some general principles helpful in diagnosing an inflamed eye:
- If the eye is only slightly pink, the pupils equal, and the eyelids matted together on awakening, the patient probably has acute conjunctivitis.
- If only one eye is inflamed, but the pupils are equal, the condition is probably innocuous. Unequal pupils may indicate serious ocular involvement.
- If the pupil is dilated, and the eye red and very painful, suspect glaucoma and call in an ophthalmologist.
- If the pupil is small, and the eye photophobic and painful, suspect iritis and, again, consult an ophthalmologist. Corneal ulceration, foreign body, or any inflammatory intraocular involvement may also cause redness of the eye and smallness of the pupil.
- If you see blood in the anterior chamber, especially after a contusion, it is a serious prognostic sign and you should consult a specialist.

Standard Management

Expectant treatment for any inflammatory ocular condition, in the absence of signs suggesting referral or until positive diagnosis is made, should consist only of broad-range local antibiotics. These include chloramphenicol, tetracycline, oxytetracycline, bacitracin, neomycin, and others, alone or in various combinations that are available commercially as eyedrops or ointments. Ointment is ordinarily reserved for bedtime use to help prevent the lashes from matting together during sleep. Drops are preferable during the day because they do not cause blurring of vision as ointment does when it melts and forms a film. Steroids must be avoided and are especially contraindicated in virus infections. The great increase in severe keratitis due to herpes simplex that has spread into the corneal stroma is attributed to the promiscuous use of steroids during the acute phase of the disease. Steroids, used with antibiotics, may also promote the growth of fungi and probably explain the increased incidence of corneal ulceration due to fungal infection.

FAILING VISION IN THE ELDERLY

One of the most tragic aspects of growing old is to experience the gradual death of the five senses. This is particularly true of *vision*, since vision is so important for pursuit of pleasure in old age — for reading and for watching television. To preserve a patient's vision, then, is to preserve his major source of happiness in old age. There are ways to do this, and I would like to tell how, by discussing some of the more common eye problems in elderly patients.

The three most common problems are macular disease, cataracts, and glaucoma. Macular disease accounts for about 45% of eye problems in the aged, cataracts account for about 33%, and glaucoma accounts for about 5%. Let us consider these disorders and several others, to see why they occur and what can be done about them.

Cataracts — When to Remove Them

Throughout a person's life, the lens of the eye grows by laying down new fibers. Simultaneously, there is a compensatory shrinkage or drying of its nucleus, which keeps it from becoming so large as to fill up the entire globe. At the same time, the lens capsule thickens and becomes less permeable. This thickening, together with hardening and drying of the nucleus and alteration of lens metabolism, progresses with age to a pathologic, disabling state where the nucleus is too hard and dry to transmit light efficiently. The cortex also becomes opaque and may become liquefied. Cataractous changes may occur in any portion of the lens, including the cortex, nucleus, and subcapsular areas. Probably everyone would acquire cataracts if he lived long enough, even though the age of onset varies widely in different individuals and families. Technically, every lens opacity is a cataract, but the condition becomes a surgical problem only when it interferes with vision.

The chief indication for surgery is when the cataract interferes with *useful* vision, and hence depends on the patient's occupation or needs.

When a patient has a cataract so advanced that you cannot evaluate the retina because of opacity, it probably should be removed. Even if

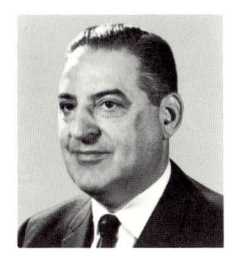

Dan M. Gordon, M.D.
Cornell University

Doctor Gordon is Associate Professor of Clinical Surgery (Ophthalmology) at Cornell University Medical College. His professional affiliations include the American College of Surgeons and the American Academy of Ophthalmology and Otolaryngology. He is Chairman Emeritus of the Scientific Advisory Council of the National Council to Combat Blindness.

the patient does have a diseased macula, removing the cataractous lens may give him better peripheral vision and make it possible for him to read with the use of magnification. However, the ophthalmologist you consult may hesitate to remove an advanced cataract in one eye when the patient has useful vision in the other. This is because an eye from which a lens has been removed cannot function in teamwork with the other eye with ordinary spectacles. The only lens that will permit the operated eye to function in binocular single vision with the unoperated eye is a contact lens, and it is difficult to get older people to go to the "trouble" of learning how to use contact lenses.

On the other hand, many ophthalmologists will advise the elderly patient with two cataracts to have only one removed, since this should suffice to give him useful vision. Theoretically, this is good reasoning, but in practice the patient often resents the blur caused by his unoperated eye and will ask to have the other eye operated on, too. Unfortunately, we cannot offer any treatment other than surgery for senile cataracts.

Senile Macular Degenerations

The so-called senile macular degenerations usually affect both eyes and are probably secondary to some vascular change. We are just beginning to learn more about atherosclerotic changes occurring in the retinal and choroidal vessels.

When sclerosis affects the macular region, there may be a dramatic loss of central vision. You can see the changes with an ophthalmoscope as they occur in the retinal vessels, but there is no known *specific* treatment or method of prevention. Sclerotic choroidal vessels may be visible as broad, flat, white lines lying deep in the retina. Frequently you will see white excrescences on Bruch's membrane between the retina and choroid; these are drüsen or colloid bodies: round white spots scattered mostly in and around the macula.

With advancing age, sclerosis and atrophy of the retinal neuroepithelium occur. Cystic changes in the peripheral retina may lead to formation of holes, which often are harmless, but which can produce a retinal detachment. Hole formation and retinal detachments are more common in myopia.

The central blindness produced by disease of the macula, characterized by loss of the ability to read or to make out detail, is a benign type of blindness. When sclerotic changes affect the mid-periphery and far periphery, the effect is more serious, for then the patient acquires "tunnel vision," which may be so extreme as to make it impossible for him to see the eyes or ears of a person's face when he is looking at the person's nose.

Other Sclerotic Changes

With advancing age, progressive arteriosclerotic changes in the optic nerve may produce atrophy. Vessel occlusions may occur within the optic nerve or in its nutrient supply. The pressure of sclerotic carotid arteries on the intracranial portion of the optic nerve may produce a picture that, ophthalmoscopically, resembles glaucoma and is known as cavernous optic atrophy. This produces bizarre visual-field changes. The extraocular nerves may be affected in the elderly, especially those with diabetes or high blood pressure. The resultant nerve palsies most often involve either the medial or lateral rectus muscles. Aneurysms of the circle of Willis also cause eye muscle palsies.

Spots Before the Eyes

One of the most prominent ocular complaints, starting at about the age of 40 or 50, is that of spots before the eyes. These are usually due to benign degenerative changes in the vitreous; they are annoying, but are otherwise insignificant. The spots may also be caused by small vitreous hemorrhages, and the complaint warrants careful investigation because it can also be associated with retinal detachment, a serious condition.

Large vitreous hemorrhages, which are more common in diabetic and, occasionally, hypertensive patients, obscure vision, but fortunately they have a high incidence of spontaneous resolution. These, too, warrant thorough investigation, for a large vitreous hemorrhage often masks retinal detachment.

Glaucoma – An Important Senile Change

Glaucoma is one of the most important senile changes. This disorder exists in many forms: acute glaucoma, chronic wide-angle (the most common form), and chronic narrow-angle glaucoma. It may be secondary to other ocular diseases, such as uveitis and tumors. The chance that a patient will have glaucoma increases markedly with age, for about 90% of all cases occur in patients more than 40 years old.

I feel that, because of the increased medical awareness of the problem and of the need for early diagnosis, there will be a marked decrease in the incidence of visual disability due to glaucoma in the years to come. Complaints of transient blurring of vision, glasses looking "dirty" when they are not, halos around lights, and the need for frequent refractions should lead you to suspect glaucoma. A patient with these complaints, especially if he is past 40 years of age, should be examined by tonometry.

Managing Senile Ocular Disorders

Most of our elderly patients have useful vision, and may require only good refraction for improvement. Those who do not, however, need more specialized medical care. The most important disabling eye diseases — cataracts, the glaucomas, macular disease, and vascular disease — require the combined efforts of family physicians and ophthalmologists for early diagnosis and proper management.

We are all familiar with the case of the grandmother whose vision has been poor and then suddenly becomes good enough for her to read again. This so-called "second sight" is usually due to increased sclerosis of the lens nucleus, which produces an artificial myopia. During this period she may even be able to read without glasses. If she dies before the sclerosis progresses to the point of opacification, she and her family may never know that she had a cataract. Often, however, her vision will fail again and not return until the diseased lens is removed.

If a cataract is removed and a macular lesion is then discovered, central vision will be markedly impaired but may be facilitated by the use of low-vision aids. When there is a central corneal scar and a cataract is to be removed, the ophthalmologist will attempt to create a new pupil around the scar.

One of the bright spots of the last decade has been the introduction of new and improved medications for the treatment of glaucoma. While none of these solves the problem by curing the disease, all facilitate its control. The newer medications, such as acetazolamide, dichlorphenamide, ethoxzolamide, and the newer miotics, have markedly decreased the number of patients with chronic glaucoma who need surgery, and have improved their prognosis for useful visual life.

The various diseases and degenerations of the macula are progressive. When they are inflammatory, they may respond to systemic and subconjunctival administration of the various corticosteroids, which often mitigate macular scarring when employed early and intensively. Some patients with senile macular degeneration *without* any inflammatory component have responded to systemic corticosteroids. I doubt that the drugs have any effect on the degenerative condition; they probably function by removing fluid from the diseased retina. Regardless of their mechanism of action, they should be given a trial of a month or two in patients with macular degeneration.

Vascular diseases and accidents, frequently related to systemic disease, are often responsible for visual disability. Ophthalmologists seem to be about evenly divided between those who do and those who do not employ anticoagulant therapy in patients who have had venous occlusions. I feel that when a patient has a branch block or a central vein occlusion, he should be offered the benefit of anticoagulant and fibrinolytic therapy. It is too early to say what effect fibrinolytic therapy has on retinal vessel occlusion; perhaps it will prove more effective if introduced directly into the carotids. Immediately after an arterial occlusion, sudden decompression of the globe by medical or surgical means (anterior-chamber puncture) and the simultaneous use of a good vasodilator such as amyl nitrite may save the eye. There have been reports of vision restored, after arterial and venous occlusion, with the use of the newer thrombolytic agents that employ fibrinolysin.

In patients complaining of transient blurring of vision, ophthalmodynamometry is indicated.

Conjunctivitis

Conjunctivitis is an important condition in the aged, because their threshold for pain is markedly lowered. The use of a mild ocular decongestant, such as tetrahydrozoline, 0.05%, or a topical steroid often brings great relief. When a truly infected conjunctivitis occurs, it should be treated with a suitable topical antibiotic.

You will be able to help many of your elderly patients by the simple suggestion that they use one of an increasing variety of low-vision aids. These magnifying devices, which are used either as hand-held magnifiers or incorporated into spectacle lenses, will make the lives of many elderly patients fuller by enabling them to read.

chapter 5

COMPLAINTS ABOUT THE MIND AND EMOTIONS

CRIPPLING ANXIETY

The patient who needs your help for anxiety suffers from an excess of one of the most crippling human emotions. To laymen, anxiety means a feeling of uneasiness, apprehension, or dread. To physicians, anxiety means not just a feeling, but something total: the heart beats faster, blood sugar rises, clotting time decreases, gaseous exchanges are affected, muscles tense, attention sharpens but narrows, and sometimes memory is blocked.

To psychiatrists it means all this and more. While the exact nature of anxiety remains controversial, most psychiatrists would agree on the following fundamental concepts. We view anxiety as an inevitable part of life, indeed essential to the growth of the personality. In unfamiliar situations, healthy people are anxious because they recognize their human vulnerability and their limited capabilities, yet they courageously overcome or at least endure threats, both external and internal, without losing their sense of identity. By sense of identity, we mean that the self is viewed as a unified whole — separate yet involved in normal relationships with others, maintaining an interest in life and the struggle it demands, retaining a sense of self-worth, and realistically assessing one's abilities. In contrast, the neurotic person, when he becomes anxious, is quite unable to maintain his goals and purposes. His efficiency is progressively reduced and indeed may be totally lost by his need to protect himself against anxiety. He may develop obsessive-compulsive defenses or become extremely dependent or completely passive and "do nothing" so that he will not get into any trouble, or he may even develop an amnesia to block out what he cannot stand. As an alternative way of dealing with anxiety, he may run away (actually), or he may simply give up and withdraw from a problem. But no matter what he does, the neurotic person always finds his efficiency decreased; he becomes fatigued; he cannot deal with extra loads, no matter how small; he cannot sleep as well; he cannot eat as well; he cannot concentrate adequately; he cannot make decisions. He is a person trying to do two things at the same time — struggle with his anxiety and maintain his ordinary dealings with reality — and does neither very well.

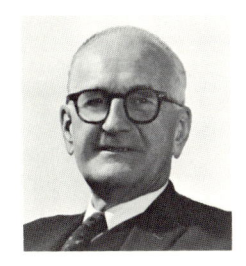

D. Ewen Cameron, M.D.
McGill University

Doctor Cameron is Chairman of the Department of Psychiatry of McGill University Faculty of Medicine, Psychiatrist-in-Chief of the Royal Victoria Hospital, and Director of the Allan Memorial Institute in Montreal. He is President of the World Psychiatric Association and a past president of the American Psychiatric Association. He received the Adolf Meyer Award in 1957 and is a Fellow of the Royal College of Physicians and Surgeons (Canada).

Such a brief outline of the psychiatric concept of anxiety is necessarily oversimplified, but perhaps it will help you anyway; you do not need to understand detailed psychiatric theory to diagnose or treat anxiety in everyday practice. Indeed, the only reason for including this much theory is to put the following rather superficial explanation of anxiety into perspective.

Anxiety is a normal response to danger, real or imaginary; for instance, being lost in the woods, being in a skidding car, anticipating a devastating job interview, or being asked to speak in public. You, as a physician, probably experience anxiety when your patients are in danger.

The boundary line between normal and abnormal anxiety is somewhat difficult to define but, in general, anxiety is abnormal when it defeats its own purpose, when it is so intense that it impairs a person's ability to deal with the emergency. It is also abnormal when the cause is trivial (fearing crowded places) or really not threatening (fearing a dead bird). It is abnormal when defenses against it are crippling. For example, to escape intolerable anxiety a woman may have to concentrate full attention on doing everything precisely, returning home to double-check, perhaps triple-check, that the taps are turned off, that the doors are locked. Again we see it in the man who must always depend on others and, for this reason, can never assert himself.

How to Recognize Anxiety

Often, recognition is easy. The patient may say he feels nervous and tense, that he has butterflies in his stomach, that he is afraid to go into crowded places, and so forth. Or he may say that without reason he has attacks, times when things seem intensely frightening, when familiar things lose their familiarity. He may fear that he will lose control of himself, that some dreadful thing will happen, or that he is about to die.

Objectively, you can usually recognize that a person is anxious by the way he talks or what he does. He says, "One can't be too careful; things are sure to go wrong." He runs to his doctor with every little complaint; he interprets his boss's every glance as a sign of dissatisfaction and possible dismissal. What he says tells a great deal; *how he says it* tells even more: the low tones, the shaky voice, the curious roughness of voice characteristic of one emotionally disturbed. Apart from the voice, nonverbal communication shows itself in posture and in movement: restless hands drumming on the table, agitated rocking, pacing the floor.

Of course, a few people can control their expression and their actions, so that they can smile even in the depths of anxiety. But they cannot control the physiologic changes caused by anxiety: sweating of the hands and feet, sweating on the upper lip, dilation of the pupils, increased respiration, and rapidity of the pulse.

Why the Anxiety?

Recognizing the signs of anxiety is not difficult, but recognizing the causes may be. Of course, they sometimes lie right on the surface and can be uncovered by a question or two. Perhaps the mother-in-law is interfering with the management of the children. Perhaps there is a new boss who is driving the patient beyond his ability, or perhaps he is pushing himself too hard. Simpler still: perhaps the patient has had a coronary attack, and has been told by someone — not necessarily his doctor — that he has only months to live.

Also, many too-much-for-too-long situations may evoke anxiety; the long-continued friction in the home or the day-in, day-out pressures on the housewife may eventually evoke anxiety. The mother with a premature child who must be fed every two hours, the parents of a delinquent child, the mother of a mentally retarded child — all are common examples. Other causes of anxiety may be hidden deeper: early lack of mother love, profound feelings of inadequacy caused by early sibling rivalry, unconscious homosexual urges, the emergence of aggressive impulses in an outwardly friendly person, and so forth.

Dealing with Anxiety

Because anxiety is as old as man, people long ago worked out ways of dealing with it. They (1) escape in flight, (2) try to build up strength to meet the threat, or (3) try to blunt the response. Let us take these human ways of dealing with anxiety and see how you can apply them.

First, as soon as you recognize that the cause of a patient's anxiety is a continuing thing, look for ways to remove her from it. Obviously, you can reduce the wife's anxiety about her interfering mother-in-law by trying to get the mother-in-law to live elsewhere. Of course, the old lady's tenacity or the husband's determination to have two women competing for him may block such direct action, so let us consider more subtle ways of separating the patient from the threat. Self-knowledge sometimes helps. For instance, the tense bank teller who sets himself impossibly high standards may, in a single interview, understand himself and lower his standards. Or the housewife who works as a secretary while she tries to keep her home neat as a pin may be able to change her ways. But then, on the other hand, she may not; she may sometimes continue to drive herself, impelled by an identification with her father, for instance, a man who also worked day and night and extolled those who did. To uncover and correct life-long attitudes such as this usually requires referral for psychotherapy.

The second great human response to anxiety, attempting to augment one's own strength to meet the threat, is done every day — for example, when we talk out our fears with someone. When two people talk together, their confidence is increased. This is especially effective when a patient talks to his physician, someone who knows how the body works, who has seen much of life. Psychotherapy differs from just talk only in that the patient's identification with the doctor goes further. He sees his anxiety through his doctor's eyes; once he learns, for example, that his inadequacy stems from past dominance by his father or from possessive overprotection by his mother, he can gradually learn to assert himself.

Another method of augmenting strength against fear is *doing something about it, acting*. A person who fears speaking in public, for example, and fears it because it means a threat to his poise and confidence, may work to improve his skill: he may enroll in speech courses or force himself to join discussion groups. By training and study, he may overcome his real inadequacies; by actually speaking before an audience, he may overcome his unrealistic fears.

If the incentive is great enough, a person may devise effective ways of conquering the fear. I know of one woman who had a life-long fear of going into water. When her family purchased a motorboat and water-skiing equipment, and she saw how much fun they had, she mustered enough courage to put on a life belt one day, ride out to the middle of a lake, and plunge into the water so that she could water-ski. Direct combat by action is an effective means of overcoming anxiety.

Finally, the third way in which man has attempted to reduce paralyzing anxiety is by limiting his responses. Down through the centuries he has depended primarily upon alcohol to do this, but in the last few decades he has discovered safer, more efficient chemicals, sedatives, and tranquilizers. Combinations of sodium amytal (65 mg.) and chlorpromazine (25 mg.) three times a day are exceedingly useful. The long list of drugs, from meprobamate to chlordiazepoxide hydrochloride, is familiar to you and you probably use them effectively, but they do not by any means comprise all the ways we have of curbing excessive anxiety. An interesting hospital procedure: administering increasing doses of insulin, from an initial dose of 5 units to not more than 60 units a day, depending on the patient's response. The patient passes into hypoglycemia for about 2 hours, without loss of consciousness; he then eats a high-carbohydrate meal. The procedure is repeated daily some 20 or 30 times. Still other methods include the "abreactive procedures": giving intravenous sodium amytal and dextroamphetamine or, in a hospital, giving nitrous oxide or ether inhalations every second day for 2 or 3 weeks. All these techniques break up anxiety reaction patterns by producing intense but controlled reactions; the day-to-day level of anxiety is thereby progressively reduced.

PATHOLOGICAL DEPRESSION
Diagnostic Clues

The young housewife appeared tired as she sank into my office chair. Moments passed before she said, "I guess I'm sort of embarrassed coming to you, Doctor. Our family doctor has managed to keep me pretty well most of the time, but lately I've been sick and I guess he's given up on me. He insisted that I come to you, and I suppose that means he thinks it's all in my mind or something."

"Well, Mrs. Forbes, I've talked to your doctor and he hasn't given up at all. He's going to direct your treatment, but he wants someone else to look at these things from a different angle. Tell me about your present troubles."

She smiled wanly, sighed deeply and put her hands on the sides of her chest. "I suppose the back pains are the worst. The thought of food nauseates me, and I don't sleep nights. I'm about to drive my husband daffy. When I have my period I go to bed for two days and everything seems so — well — that's the worst time of all, and the children just about drive me out of my mind . . ."

Mrs. Forbes is depressed. There may be an underlying physical disorder, but whether or not there is organic pathology, she is depressed enough to need treatment for it. And this is a type of depression her family physician can treat medically. Indeed, this type of depression is one of the most common disorders seen by the family physician, who can now treat (symptomatically) most nonpsychotic depressions about as well as a psychiatrist. The most important step, of course, is to suspect and recognize its presence. Treatment is being discussed elsewhere in these pages, so I will talk only about making the diagnosis of depression.

Depression Is Abnormal Grief

Depression is easier understood if we think of it as simply prolonged or abnormal grief. Although it may result from obvious losses or frustrations, sometimes it is in response to losses and frustrations that are not evident either to the depressed person or to others. That is why it is

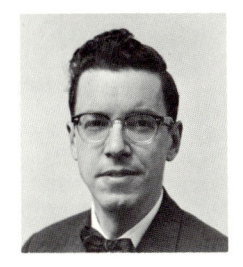

James R. Harris, M.D.
University of Pennsylvania

Doctor Harris is Executive Medical Officer of the Institute of the Hospital of Pennsylvania, and Associate Professor of Psychiatry at the University of Pennsylvania School of Medicine. He is psychiatrist and a trustee at Horizon House (Philadelphia), a rehabilitation center for former mental patients. He is certified by the National Board of Psychiatry and Neurology and is a Fellow of the American Psychiatric Association.

sometimes hard to sympathize with a chronically depressed person. We can keep saying, "Cheer up, for goodness sake! You have nothing to be depressed about." But no matter how the depressed person tries to prove he is *not* depressed, inwardly he is grieving, and it is a very real grief. He may also be angry at himself, and secretly angry at others. His grief and anger may be so strong that he commits suicide, or attempts to do so.

At the end of this article you will find a review of the various types of depression, with the characteristics of each outlined in some detail. Knowledge of the several forms in which depression appears is necessary if you are to make the right classification when you examine the patient.

Examining for Depression

Depression is similar to other diseases in this respect: to diagnose it you must first suspect its presence. Put differently, a mild depression is almost never noticed unless specifically looked for. Depression is found most often in elderly persons, in persons who have suffered recent losses or disappointments, who have chronic complaints, whether or not the complaints seem justified, who repeatedly suffer from accidents and injuries, and who have recently had a change in personality or habits, especially those who become irritable, fatigued, or who begin to take sedatives or alcohol excessively. Depression can, however, appear at any age, even in young children.

During the routine examination of a patient, the following areas should be explored carefully.

General Appearance

The depressed patient appears quieter than usual and slower in his movements. His muscle tonus is frequently reduced, and he walks in a stooped, tired manner, his chest sunken. His facial muscles sag a bit, so that he appears older than his age, and even when he forces a smile he has a hangdog expression with a somewhat glassy or vacant stare. His speech is slow and his voice reveals little emotion. He may try to cover this over with forced cheerfulness, but if you catch him unaware he will usually have resumed his depressed manner and appearance.

Content of Conversation

The depressed patient talks mostly about his past, views the future with pessimism bordering on the hopeless. This is one of the most important diagnostic features and should be brought out by gentle but specific questions. You might ask, "How do you think things will turn out?" or,

"What are your future plans?" Sometimes the patient will announce spontaneously, "The future is absolutely black. I can see nothing ahead but failure and defeat." More frequently, though, he will avoid such direct statements and hint at despair, or he will become noticeably sad and pessimistic when talking about future plans. Such remarks as, "I guess this pain will go on forever," or "I just know I'll get worse and worse," are quite common. The patient's attitude may also be expressed by such remarks as, "Thanks for trying, Doctor, but it's no use. You might as well tell me the worst." However, when the past is brought up, the depressed person becomes more willing to talk, to remember specific details, and when talking about his childhood he sometimes appears comforted and relieved. If asked when was the happiest time of his life, he usually picks a time when he was very young and dependent.

Depressed persons are also very self-centered in their conversations. It is difficult to get them off the subject of themselves. They dwell endlessly on their pains, suffering and misfortunes. They talk of how they have sacrificed, how they have sinned, the mistakes they have made, and give an impression that things will never change. They often go into detail about habits of urination, defecation, coughing, heartbeat, digestion, sleeping and eating habits. Interspersed between these remarks is the frequent, "I don't see how anyone can put up with me; I'm such a burden and nuisance."

Disturbances of Thinking

In involutional and psychotic depressions, but rarely in reactive depressions, paranoid thinking becomes prominent. There are often delusions of reference (People are looking at me; messages are being sent to me over television; the White House is talking about me), and delusions of persecution (My wife is poisoning me; the FBI is following me; the neighbors are whispering lies about me), and delusions of bodily change (My blood is rotting; my liver is shrinking; my intestines are closing off). Occasionally a doubting of reality occurs (Things aren't real; I'm not really me). Thinking may become slowed, and this will be evident in the repetitious or stereotyped answers to your questions, as if the patient is stalling to collect his lagging thoughts. In agitated depressions, thinking may become repetitive, with the same disturbing thought racing through the brain for hours.

Physical Symptoms

There are few specific physical symptoms in reactive depressions, although it must be remembered that depressions often occur with organic disorders of all types. Severe psychotic depressions may show obstipation, dry skin, low blood pressure, slowed pulse, decreased muscle tonus, lessened salivation and tearing, skin and corneal ulcers, pneumonia, marked weight loss, avitaminosis, and in extreme cases stupor or endless agitation leading to exhaustion.

When dealing with depression, remember that (1) it is among the most common disorders seen by doctors today, (2) it is a symptomatic diagnosis only, and it may have several etiologies, (3) it often accompanies organic illness, but may come disguised in a wide variety of somatic complaints, (4) nonpsychotic depressions can be treated medically, and the prognosis is good if they are recognized and treated early.

*   *   *

Types of Depression

NORMAL GRIEF may be delayed a few days following a profound loss, but once it starts it begins to lessen within a short time and the person should be fully recovered within six months. If grieving is unduly prolonged, it often turns into pathological depression. Remember, however, that depression may also begin without evidence of any apparent reason for grief or frustration.

REACTIVE DEPRESSION. This type is seen most often by the family physician and is something that he can treat medically. The patient may cover his distress and appear to be happy, or he may be obviously sad, but in either case he is able to continue his life pattern more or less as usual. His *mental* symptoms may include feelings of hopelessness and worthlessness, and a general loss of initiative. He may have vague feelings that he has sinned or that he has been a bad influence on others. He tends to blame things on himself, to be passive and compliant, and occasionally irritable. Frequently, he complains of physical symptoms that either mask or accompany depression. These symptoms frequently involve a slowing down of bodily functions: metabolism, tonus, digestion and excretion. The paravertebral muscles become loose, the patient slumps over somewhat, and in trying to compensate for this he may develop back pains, headaches, vague aches in the legs. He may complain of anorexia, constipation, nausea, dizziness (orthostatic hypotension), and loss of sexual interest or sexual potency. A very important symptom can be an intensification of an existing organic illness. An arthritic patient, for example, who could put up with his pains under medication may find them becoming intolerable as he becomes depressed. Whenever an existing illness produces symptoms that are exaggerated or prolonged, depression must be suspected.

PSYCHOTIC DEPRESSION is usually readily recognized, because the patient is so afflicted that his entire life pattern must change. Thoughts of sinfulness and worthlessness dominate his mental life, and a single thought may repeat itself over and over again for hours. He feels doomed, has no hope. He speaks in a monotone or not at all. His head is bent, his stare is glassy. He suffers extreme anorexia, constipation, and even dryness of the mouth, and absence of tears. He becomes either very restless, pacing nervously, or descends into somnolent stupor. As these disturbances progress, he loses weight and may develop secondary skin or lung infections.

INVOLUTIONAL DEPRESSION. As men and women enter the so-called involutional period of their lives they become aware of their loss of youthful vigor, fertility or potency, and ambition. They become sensitive to failures and disappointments. They also undergo involutional changes in their endocrines. As a result of these real and imagined losses, they may become depressed, sometimes to extreme degrees. This type of depression is more common in females, and in persons who have always been conscientious, scrupulous, demanding, rigid and moralistic, and unable to adequately express their anger. They usually have lived successful, though restricted, lives until they reach their forties and fifties, at which time their adjustment mechanisms fail and the meaning of life seems to disappear for them. They become morose, are tortured by feelings of sinfulness, and sometimes they have bizarre delusions, extreme restlessness, and irresistible suicidal urges. In the early stages this disorder can be confused with reactive depression, but as it progresses it is readily diagnosed.

MANIC-DEPRESSIVE DISEASE is found classically in those persons subject to rhythmic changes in mood. They have a history of fluctuating states ranging from ebullient, grandiose self-satisfaction to profound discouragement and disappointment. They are usually warm, outgoing people who seem to be ruled by their passions, and when they become psychotic, they swing from wild mania or hypomania to deep depression.

DEPRESSION AS A SYMPTOM OF ORGANIC DISEASES. Chronic debilitating or infectious diseases, such as tuberculosis and cancer, are sometimes ushered in or accompanied by prolonged depressions, mild or severe.

PATHOLOGICAL DEPRESSION
Pointers About Treatment

Lately we have been seeing fewer patients with full-blown depressions in our psychiatric clinics and hospitals, which means, I believe, that family physicians are doing a superior job of recognizing and treating the predisposing neuroses. But even while paying tribute to your proficiency, I must add that neither family physicians nor psychiatrists have any reason to be smug about their handling of depression itself. Not while more than 20,000 people commit suicide each year.

But before discussing better handling of depression, I want to offer a suggestion for earlier diagnosis. You as family physicians sometimes have a unique opportunity to make a diagnosis even before the appearance of symptoms of full-blown depression.

Take this not-so-hypothetical case: Mrs. Jones, age 38, has visited you for five years. Each month or so, you listen to complaints about her hypochondriacal symptoms and her unsympathetic husband (the latter seemingly the most distressing). Each month sympathy, reassurance, and occasional tranquilizing drugs have helped her achieve a stable emotional adjustment that permits her to function passably well. Then one day she surprises you by doubting aloud that her unhappiness is the result of her husband's unloving and unwarranted actions, by wondering if she might not be deficient as a wife. But this is no time to give thanks for improved insight; this first failure of her stabilizing neurotic adjustment is quite likely the first sign of oncoming depression. So always beware of the sharp changes in the patient's way of coping with anxiety.

Directive Treatment Is Helpful

But how should you proceed once you have recognized early depression? You must try to rebuild the sense of security that has been eroded by environmental stress. Allow Mrs. Jones to escape from the stresses she faces by becoming temporarily dependent upon you. Say something like this: "Mrs. Jones, you are suffering from severe fatigue. Your burdens have been just too much. For the next few weeks, I want you to

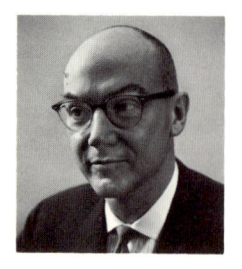

Blaine E. McLaughlin, M.D.
Woman's Medical College of Pennsylvania

Doctor McLaughlin is Associate Professor of Psychiatry and Director of the Psychiatric Service at Woman's Medical College of Pennsylvania. He is also President and Medical Director of the Medical Research Foundation of Philadelphia and a Chief of Psychiatry at Philadelphia General Hospital. He is a Diplomate of the American Board of Psychiatry and Neurology.

leave all your worries to me. I'll do everything necessary to insure your recovery. All you have to do is follow my instructions without question or exception."

Instruct her to get up at a certain hour, have breakfast at a certain hour, spend an hour and a half in physical activity during the forenoon, take a nap after lunch, spend two hours shopping with someone else in the afternoon, and fill her evening with simple escapist diversions like reading and television. Later, when she feels more secure, try to interest her in creative activities (in middle age, the less competitive ones are best), and independence will gradually return. But for now, you make the decisions.

Enlist Aid for the Supportive Program

Try to involve at least one of the patient's relatives in the supportive program (and perhaps a clergyman, parent, employer, friend or neighbor, too). For medicolegal reasons, somebody near the patient must be aware of the possibility of suicide. It also helps to impress the family with the importance of helping the patient rather than continuing the quarrelsome discordance that may have characterized the household.

Prescribe moderate doses of one of the antidepressant drugs and, if the patient is sufficiently agitated to warrant it, a tranquilizing drug also. For insomnia, you may prescribe a soporific drug, but always less than a lethal amount. Usually I prescribe a week's supply and never allow renewals. Have her return for another visit in three or four days, never longer than one week.

If treatment is to succeed, your patient must believe you know more about her condition than she does. If she finds it increasingly easy to submit to your authority, she is definitely on the mend. And the more she accepts authority, the less arbitrary and more reasonable it can become. But if she fights authority, she is slipping into a psychotic adjustment and, within one to three months, will probably have to be hospitalized.

Age Helps Determine Treatment

The treatment routine need be modified only a little when dealing with a patient other than middle-aged. Consider, for example, the college boy who was your patient during his high-school years. Besides caring for his football injuries, you were called upon to help hold him down when he seemed bent on killing himself and wrecking the community in a youthful attempt to find outlets for his seemingly boundless energy. Now, at age 20, he wants to quit college. His customary aggressive optimism is replaced by self-doubt — perhaps because of perfectionistic attitudes of his parents. The problem is *not* that he lacks the capacity for further aggressive responses but that he has not learned how to apply aggression and what results to expect. This sudden turnabout is likely to be the first sign of depression.

Again adopt an authoritarian attitude. If necessary, get him to drop a course. Try to persuade perfectionistic relatives or professors that, at least for now, they must expect less from your patient. And try to substitute your own more realistic, more human goals and standards.

By contrast, the emotional change that precedes depression is harder to detect in the elderly. The first sign seems to be gradually deepening physiologic retardation. Aunt Helen in the back bedroom is depressed because she cannot adjust to a dependent role and is too old to escape into creative activities that satisfy the middle-aged patient. Agitated depression in the elderly is often treated with too much sedation. Instead, prescribe moderate doses of antidepressants with vitamins and tonics. Even more so than in the middle-aged, you must take complete responsibility for the elderly patient. Often you can modify relatives' attitudes and improve her environment, but the best adjustment is achieved by those oldsters who gracefully regress into dependency and derive satisfaction from the achievements of younger people.

Learn to Use the New Drugs

Office management of depression has changed greatly in the past four years since the new antidepressant drugs have become available. Now the target symptoms of depression (despondency, guilt, psychomotor retardation, feelings of hopelessness and worthlessness, loss of interest and initiative, and self-reproach) can be modified by drugs in most patients.

Indeed, these drugs are so important in office treatment of depression that you need to become familiar with them just as you became familiar with the various tranquilizers ten years ago. They are no more difficult nor less safe to use than the major tranquilizers. Moreover, becoming familiar with them is not too difficult because only six different preparations are now used extensively as major antidepressant drugs; five of the six can be classified into two groups according to their mode of action.

Three are classified as monoamine oxidase inhibitors: isocarboxazid, phenelzine, and nialamide. (See Table 1.) By inhibiting MAO, they retard the breakdown of serotonin and norepinephrine in the brain, which presumably accounts for their antidepressant effect. Because their action is indirect (i.e., through enzyme metabolism), the effect may not be noticeable for one to four weeks. Liver damage, noted with the earliest drugs in this family, is rare in the newer ones; indeed it has never been reported

TABLE 1 — SIX FREQUENTLY USED ANTIDEPRESSANT DRUGS

Generic Name	Trade Name	Recommended Dosage (mg/day)*		
		Starting	Maintenance	Maximum
MAO INHIBITORS				
isocarboxazid	Marplan®	30	10-20	30
phenelzine	Nardil®	45	15-45	75
nialamide	Niamid®	75-100	variable	200
NON-MAO INHIBITORS				
imipramine	Tofrānil®	75†	50-150†	200†
amitriptyline	Elavil®	75	40-150	150
meprobamate + benactyzine	Deprol®	1 tablet q.i.d.**	1 tablet q.i.d.**	1 tablet q.i.d.**

* According to manufacturers' listings in PHYSICIANS' DESK REFERENCE TO PHARMACEUTICAL SPECIALTIES AND BIOLOGICALS, ed. 18, Oradell, N. J., Medical Economics, Inc., 1964. Since manufacturers' recommendations change from time to time, current literature should be consulted before these drugs are prescribed.

† For all outpatients except geriatric and adolescent.
** 1,600 mg. meprobamate plus 4 mg. benactyzine.

with nialamide.

Two other drugs, imipramine and amitriptyline, apparently achieve their antidepressant effect by suppressing the subcortical structures of the central nervous system. Some of their beneficial and side effects resemble those of the phenothiazine tranquilizers, to which they are chemically related. For example, unlike the MAO inhibitors, they are more likely to sedate than overstimulate your patient. The antidepressant effects of these two suppressants are also slow to appear. The sixth frequently used antidepressant preparation is a combination of two tranquilizers, meprobamate and benactyzine.

Naturally, before using any of the six drugs, you should read carefully the doses, indications, and cautions listed by their manufacturers. In this short article I can only say that they are *relatively* potent, safe drugs. Certainly the danger of their causing serious side effects is less than allowing even a "mild" depression to go untreated.

Nor can I tell you which drug is more likely to benefit a particular patient. Even those clinicians most familiar with these drugs usually select by trial and error. They first use the drug they have become most familiar with; then they switch to another if adequate trial proves the first choice ineffective (being careful to allow a medication-free week to pass when switching from imipramine or amitriptyline to the incompatible MAO inhibitors or vice versa). And always remember, at the first sign of serious depression or suicidal intent, refer for hospitalization and perhaps electroshock therapy, which remains one of the most effective treatments of all.

IMAGINARY ILLS

Few of us like the patient with imaginary ills — the hypochondriac. We refer to him contemptuously among ourselves as a "crock." We consider him the bane of medical practice to be mollified or passed on to some zealous newcomer as quickly as possible. However, our irritation with him may reflect our lack of understanding of him and his illness.

What Is Hypochondriasis?

Hypochondriasis is often a wastebasket category, used to cover everything from simple preoccupation with somatic symptoms to the extreme delusional convictions of somatic harm. In this paper, I will use H. R. Laughlin's restricted definition: "an obsessive kind of preoccupation with physical symptoms or body processes which is often accompanied by the development of various, and often shifting, somatic complaints." Characteristically, these patients are overdemanding and irritably persistent in their illness, they complain of an inappropriate degree of somatic discomfort, and they take satisfaction in their illness and pleasure in foiling your efforts to cure them. They usually show a *need* for their symptoms as a solution for some life difficulty.

The Need to Be Sick

The symptoms of hypochondriasis serve a set of unconscious needs and purposes. Perhaps the foremost need is the assuagement of guilt, usually unconsciously repressed. There are mechanisms by which unconscious or irrational guilt are produced: First, the infantile mind is unable to differentiate between thinking a thing and doing a thing; i.e., it holds itself equally culpable for the thought as for the deed. Another mechanism is a primitive, logical fallacy that prompts a conclusion of causal link between a wish or deed and subsequent events. For example, if a parent dies, a child unconsciously considers that his evil thoughts or death wishes caused the death, and that he is therefore responsible, as a murderer. He feels guilty, and because guilt is so painful and unaccept-

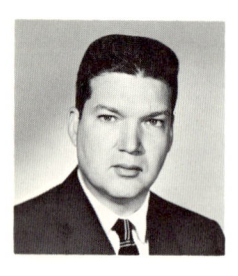

Charles W. Wahl, M.D.
University of California, Los Angeles

Doctor Wahl is Associate Professor and Chief of the Division of Psychosomatic Medicine, Department of Psychiatry, University of California School of Medicine. He is Consultant in Psychiatry at Sepulveda Veterans Administration Hospital and Camarillo and Metropolitan State Hospital, all near Los Angeles. He is a Diplomate of the American Board of Psychiatry and Neurology, and a member of the American Psychiatric Association.

able, it is repressed. Even so, the "crime" continues to demand expiation. The guilt of a crime, actual or fantasied, is alleviated by similar suffering; hence, the patient may have symptoms similar to those of the ambivalently loved person who died.

Whatever the symptoms, only suffering alleviates unconscious guilt. Therefore, when the hypochondriac says that he feels bad, he is often describing a state of guilt though he may be unaware of it. This partly accounts for the reluctance of the hypochondriac to surrender his physical symptoms; he unconsciously believes that as long as he suffers he is protected from a more dreaded punishment. I am reminded of the species of lizard which, when caught by a bird of prey, has the happy faculty of snapping off his wriggling tail, which the distracted predator then seizes and eats, allowing the lizard to escape and grow another.

Another mechanism is related to the above, namely, that illness may be, by unconscious logic, a defense against the fear of death. It is as if the hypochondriac remembers the parallel religious custom, that only the sheep without blemish is taken from the flock to be sacrificed; the damaged one lives on. The protective value of illness frequently appears to operate in the psychodynamics of the hypochondriac.

Another causal mechanism is the employment of illness as an expression of inadequacy. Hypochondriacs are usually people who have been reared in an atmosphere of illness by parents who make much of physical complaints. It is hard for a child to feel stronger than he perceives his parents as being. These patients, like their parents, grow up thinking of their bodies as being frail mechanisms, not equal to the tasks life assigns.

Still another mechanism is the use of an illness as the symbolic substitute for some unconscious need or unacceptable feeling. Many idioms in our language are examples of unconscious connection between emotional and somatic response. These idioms may have diagnostic significance. Patients who suffer from cervical dystonia may be forced to endure people who are "pains in the neck." Patients who suffer from epigastric nausea and distress are made "sick to their stomachs" by someone or something. Things "get under my skin," "people won't get off my back"; people with hysterical paralysis of the hands and legs may be vicariously expressing things they "can't handle" or "can't stand." Documented clinical examples by the score demonstrate that the mind and body may work together in this literally insane way.

The last mechanism is the secondary gain that illness affords, for illness achieves advantages for the patient just as deformity does for the professional beggar. It enables the patient to "fail with honor," to get sympathy and consideration, or achieve an importance otherwise unattainable. The secondary gains can often be very subtle and are not easily identified except by careful scrutiny of the patient's life situation.

The secondary gains are also usually unconscious, and you must be careful about confronting the patient with the advantages that his illness brings him.

Treatment in Your Practice

How can these patients best be treated? It depends on the degree of illness. Severe hypochondriasis may presage a severe psychiatric decompensation, so you should be on the lookout for hypochondriacal symptoms that (a) become more bizarre or changeable, (b) do not limit but intensify anxiety or depression, or (c) are associated with other neurotic symptoms. Patients with these signs had best be referred for psychiatric consultation.

But you can treat simple hypochondriasis by attempting to do the following:

- Listen to the patient. The patient has gone to the trouble to develop physical symptoms rather than complain. Now encourage him to express his feelings verbally rather than with his body. A *willingness* to listen, rather than just to listen, is what the patient wants and needs. As soon as he is assured of this, his need for an unreasonable amount of your time will be greatly diminished.
- These patients, more than any others, need a dependable confidence in you. You take the place of the parent, and this repairs the deficit in good parental relationship that is almost always the antecedent of his symptoms.
- Listen carefully to what the patient says, particularly to his idiomatic expressions. These will give you clues to the people and situations that trouble him and the fears or wishes his symptoms may symbolically displace and represent.
- Do not equivocate about your diagnosis nor hedge by suggesting alternate fearful possibilities. If you have doubts, keep them to yourself.
- Do not overstudy the patient. These patients get worse during unnecessarily detailed workups. Avoid such procedures as spinals, bronchoscopies, and so forth, if at all possible.
- Give the patient proper simple physiological explanations. Do not say that his symptoms are imaginary, but do explain how tension and muscle spasm produce pain and dysfunction. Employ simile, metaphor, description, and pictorial representation (and repetition) in getting your points across.
- Encourage these patients to look at their deep feelings of fear and need. Encourage them to put them into words. Also help them to verbalize their other life problems. Help them to see that their concern about their health may be diverting their attention from other problems.
- Use medicines sparingly. These patients do poorly with them.

DISTURBANCES THAT CALL FOR PSYCHIATRIC REFERRAL

No doubt you are familiar with much of the advice that has been published in abundance concerning your approach to the treatment of patients with mental and emotional illnesses. There is certainly no shortage of articles that will tell you that you must be interested in the patient; that you must be willing to listen; that you should not attempt deep analytical probing but that you should provide supportive therapy while avoiding the temptation to do too much directive therapy; that you should never attempt any psychotherapy in patients you cannot tolerate or find irritating; that you must examine your own desires and decide whether you are really willing to do psychotherapy in the first place; and, of course, that you must not attempt to treat patients who have serious psychiatric problems that are beyond your competence. I suspect, though, that most (and probably all) general practitioners have a clear idea of their limitations in psychiatry and are only too happy to refer patients with serious problems to a psychiatrist.

But let's say you have a patient who ought to see a psychiatrist, and you've made up your mind to refer him to one. Are there still some things you, and perhaps only you, can do to help the patient? I think so, and I hope these guidelines will prove practical.

Prepare the Patient

While education has greatly reduced the stigma attached to mental illness in the lay mind, there are still many people who fear psychiatric care or to whom the need for such care connotes failure or weakness and seems shameful — hardly helpful attitudes. One of the first and most important things you can do, then, is help the patient and the psychiatrist get off on the right foot. Anything you can do to reduce a patient's fear or to motivate him to want to get well and accept treatment will be valuable. Exactly how you do this will vary from patient to patient, but just as your discussion of sex is easier and less shocking to a patient if you use scientific terms, so will your discussion of this problem be easier if you avoid emotionally charged words.

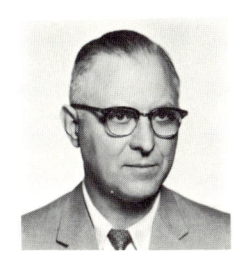

Robert L. Garrard, M.D.
Greensboro, North Carolina

Doctor Garrard is a Fellow of the American Psychiatric Association, a member of the American Academy of Neurology, and is a past president of the Guilford County Medical Association. During World War II, he served as a Lt. Colonel (MC) with the U.S. Army in the European and Pacific theatres of operation. He is currently in private practice, and his chief interests are forensic medicine and psychiatry.

To some patients, you may have to explain that mental illness can take many forms, and brief the patient on what he can expect the psychiatrist to do. It may be helpful to remind your patient of how universal the problem of mental and emotional disorders is, and emphasize that his problem is not a sign of weakness. You might add a note of flattery (depending on the patient's status, of course) by mentioning that the incidence of such problems is higher among professional and executive people than among the unskilled. Perhaps describing the improvement experienced by another patient who had a similar problem would help. It may be wise, if it is true, to reassure him that referral need not mean hospitalization.

However you choose to approach this problem, frankness is almost always better than deception. Attempts to conceal the fact that the psychiatrist *is* a psychiatrist, for example, are seldom successful and when the patient sees through the deception he almost always reacts unfavorably.

Advise the Family

The patient's family usually needs advice, too, and you are in the best position to give it. Although the cooperation of a responsible relative may be absolutely necessary only when referring severely disturbed psychotic patients, you should always explain the situation to the family as completely as circumstances will permit and enlist their support.

I realize that you may run across a frankly hostile relative to whom you should not give information that may be used against the patient, but destructive influences in the home that may negate progress in treatment are usually caused by ignorance rather than malice. It is difficult, for example, for some relatives to accept that the patient is sick and in need of treatment rather than discipline. Often, it is a troublesome home environment that precipitated the patient's breakdown in the first place, and it is of little benefit to help the patient only to re-expose him to the cause of his illness. (Occasionally, indeed, a relative may need treatment as much as the patient.) By discussing the problem with the family you may uncover and perhaps eliminate trouble spots.

You may find it helpful to recommend one of several good books on mental and emotional illness that have been written for the layman. For example:

- EMOTIONAL ILLNESS: HOW FAMILIES CAN HELP, by Beutner and Hale (Putnam, $2.50).
- MENTAL HEALTH IS A FAMILY AFFAIR, by Pratt and Neher (Public Affairs Pamphlet No. 155, 25¢).
- WHEN YOU GROW OLDER, by Lawton and Stewart (Public Affairs Pamphlet No. 131, 25¢).

Provide a Good Case History

You should provide a thorough case history, including personal information that you might not, perhaps even *should* not, send to another specialist — a surgeon, for example. Mental illness serious enough to require treatment by a psychiatrist does not develop overnight. While some single event (divorce, being fired, death of a loved one) may make the illness flare up, the basic problem has been smoldering for some time, and anything you can tell the psychiatrist about the patient's background, childhood deficiencies, family and occupational difficulties, sex problems, resentments, and so forth, will be helpful. By telling the psychiatrist at once things that might otherwise remain concealed or be disclosed by the patient only after long and searching interviews, you may contribute substantially to the value of treatment and save the patient considerable time and expense.

Referring physicians seldom fail to tell me about the socially unacceptable incidents in a patient's background: he's always getting into fights; he drinks too much; he's been unfaithful. Less frequently, though, do they tell me that a patient is too good to be true: the adolescent who never gets into trouble; the man who is always reading the Bible and goes to church every day; the model husband who never argues about anything, either in the home or out. My point is not that any of these is a definite indication of psychiatric illness, but that the extreme in either direction — "good" or "bad"—*may* be significant.

Follow up After Referral

After referral, you may encounter two problems. First, the patient may reject the psychiatrist after several visits. If this happens, try to find out why the patient has rejected him. If you cannot overcome his objections, suggest a different psychiatrist. Be sure to tell the second psychiatrist that the patient has rejected another one. Second, you may wonder what to do while the patient is seeing the psychiatrist. If the patient wants, you should continue seeing him. Ordinarily, you should limit yourself to reassuring him, and his family if necessary, and explaining the psychiatrist's reports to the family in terms they can understand. Avoid letting the patient put you in the position of contradicting the psychiatrist. If the patient tells you something about the treatment that seems unreasonable, withhold judgment until you've checked with the psychiatrist. The patient's version, after all, may be distorted, or what seems unreasonable on the surface may be reasonable once it's explained.

BED-WETTING

When bed-wetting persists beyond the age of three or four, it assumes growing importance as a problem because more often than not, it is made worse by attempts to control it. The parents often enter into a battle of wits with the child, using bribes, promises, threats, and scorn to try to induce him to control his bladder. But these efforts only magnify the problem and perpetuate the habit. What was originally a dysfunction of immaturity now becomes a disturbing chain of events that affects the child in many ways: every relationship he has may be adversely affected and, as a result, his self-esteem, in particular, and social development, in general, suffer. If you can successfully step into this battle between the parents and child, you may be able to do much to remove this roadblock to the child's healthy interpersonal development.

Enuresis Sets up a Vicious Cycle

Few parents can tolerate bed-wetting easily. Almost any mother eventually resents having to change linen frequently and constantly being reminded of the problem by the odor of urine, which clings to the child's room despite heroic scrubbings. If the child is competent in other areas of life, the parents may come to view the habit as a form of obstinate perversity. They may feel it as anger directed at them (which it frequently is) and react with counteranger. If there are other symptoms of emotional disturbance, they may feel it as reproach, testifying to their inadequacy as parents and react anxiously or perhaps punitively.

If the enuretic child has brothers and sisters, they, too, react. They may resent the additional attention he gets and express their jealousy and rivalry by taunting him in the presence of playmates. Other effects on his friendships may be even more serious: he usually avoids sleep-out dates, and hesitates to invite other children to spend the night at his home. He may even be afraid to have children play in his room, lest the odor betray him. Finally, finding himself gradually cut off from the expanding activity of his friends, frequently reminded of his affliction by the taunts of brothers and sisters, recurrently experiencing the dis-

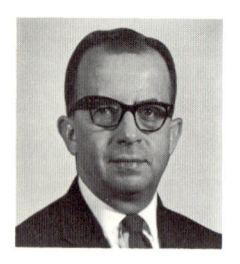

Milton Mazer, M.D.
Martha's Vineyard Guidance Center, Massachusetts

Doctor Mazer is Director of the Martha's Vineyard Guidance Center, a nonprofit agency providing individual and community psychiatric services for the residents of this island off the coast of Massachusetts. He also serves on the faculty of the William Alanson White Institute of Psychiatry, Psychoanalysis, and Psychology. He is a Diplomate of the American Board of Psychiatry and Neurology.

pleasure of one or both parents, the child will lose self-esteem, and this, of course, is the most damaging consequence of all.

The First Step in Management

In approaching the problem with the child's parents, you must first undo much of what has already been done. More than likely, they have already used many coercive and punitive measures to no avail. At the outset, you should make it clear that enuresis is not a willful disobedience but rather the result of unconscious forces which the child, at the moment, cannot control. You should help them understand that although they can control many aspects of their child's life they cannot control his bladder—only the child himself can. In any contest in this area, the struggle is an unequal one, with the child almost inevitably winning and thus *reinforcing his symptom*.

Methods based on the principle of conditioning have been widely used. You are apt to find that the parents have been advised by friends or books to wake the child during the night to take him to the toilet. This method is based on the assumption that the child's bladder overflows because it cannot hold the night's urinary output. The method may occasionally be useful in mild cases where parental cooperation is assured. In practice, however, the sleepy parent is usually understandably in a hurry to get the task over with, and, so, takes the child to the toilet and induces him to urinate when the child is not fully awake. The result is, in effect, a further conditioning of the child to *urinate while asleep*.

Electrical devices designed to awaken the child as soon as he begins to urinate—by the ringing of a bell or the flashing of a light—may occasionally be effective, if they are accepted by the child. However, they are often experienced by the child as controlling and manipulative, and he may resist them by sinking into an even deeper sleep. I know of one enuretic child who repeatedly slept through the ringing of the bell each night, while her brother would awaken and come from the adjoining room to turn it off.

Once the likelihood of organic disease of the urinary tract has been ruled out, and simple measures have failed, you can most effectively approach the problem as a disorder in interpersonal relationships. Perhaps the two most important emotional factors are anxiety and unexpressed anger.

The Anxious Child

An example of anxiety causing enuresis is the case of Betty, a 10-year-old girl I recently treated. Betty experienced a recurrence of enuresis, together with school phobia, when she was advanced ahead of her twin brother in school. I learned that Betty's mother had an excessively clinging relationship with her, and reacted anxiously to each step in Betty's growth. Betty, on her side, experienced each step forward as a *threat to her close relationship to her mother*, and when she was advanced in school ahead of her twin brother, she felt in danger of losing the nurturing of her mother. I postulated that the enuresis represented an attempt for Betty to be a little girl again and that the school phobia was a means of remaining home to guard her interests. When I discussed this possibility with both Betty and her mother, and reassured Betty that her mother would continue to be interested in her even while at school, both symptoms disappeared.

If an enuretic child has difficulty in falling asleep, and if he has some of the common fears of childhood, your approach should be directed at diminishing his fears. Frequently, such children, once they have fallen asleep, tend to sleep so soundly that they cannot be awakened easily, even by a distended bladder. If he is afraid of the dark, I suggest a night light and advise the parents to reassure the child that they are always nearby (pointing out that the door of their room is left open). If the enuresis is more or less limited to the nights preceding school days, I explore possible sources of anxiety at school. And I sometimes recommend that the parents make a point of spending a quiet time with the child in his room at bedtime, permitting him to express his fears and reassuring him.

The Angry Child

Another type of case is that of Rosalie, who at the age of 9 continued to wet the bed almost nightly. Taking her to the bathroom at intervals during the night and using a conditioning apparatus had both failed. Analysis of Rosalie's situation revealed a great deal of jealousy towards her brother, who was seventeen months younger. At this point, Rosalie's mother had an opportunity to go to England on a desirable writing assignment. This focused her attention on Rosalie's special needs, and after much reflection, she announced that she felt the child needed her too much for her to leave. Within two weeks, Rosalie's enuresis was gone.

When repressed anger is the cause of enuresis, it is often because the child feels overwhelmed by rivalry with a younger brother or sister. Since the parents are the prize of the rivalry, his anger is expressed at them. On exploring the child's daily life, you may find, as I often have, that despite the fact that he is older, the enuretic child is held to the same rules as his younger brother or sister. Since he finds no advantage in being older, he may try to use the weapon of the younger child, namely infantilism. In one case I know of, simply suggesting that the parents advance an enuretic child's bedtime 15 minutes and increase her weekly allowance by 15 cents over that of her brother was immediately followed by disappearance of the enuresis.

Above all, in treating enuresis, I believe the important thing is to apply our everyday knowledge of interpersonal relations in trying to understand the child's problem and to cope with it. When an organic cause for the disorder cannot be found, consider it as a behavioral response to disturbing problems in his interpersonal relationships—not as a symptom of a neurosis. If you can discover what these problems are, you stand a good chance of not only curing the enuresis, but also of paving the way to a healthier future for the child.

chapter 6

SLIGHT INJURIES

CUTS THAT CAN BE TREATED IN YOUR OFFICE

If you are like me, a bit frayed and frazzled, trying to maintain a regular schedule while engrossed in important and often unsolved medical problems, there is hardly anything more disconcerting than to be called on to treat the patient who has a simple laceration. These cuts yield more than their share of cusses, and yet they must be managed. Since we are all faced with this problem, perhaps there are ways of reducing the irritations and at the same time improving our technique.

Management of simple wounds tends to deteriorate in several correctible areas: (1) *poor equipment*, (2) *poor timing*, (3) *poor follow-up*, and (4) *poor diagnosis*.

To begin in the reverse order: it is certainly disconcerting to discover that what appeared to be a minor wound is, in fact, major. By definition, a simple laceration is one that does not involve important anatomic structures. Of course, size has slight relation to potential severity; oddly, the smallest wounds may be the most serious, particularly if they involve the tendons of the hand or areas of special function on the face. And, of course, the seriousness of small penetrating wounds which enter the viscera must never be underestimated.

Sensible Follow-up Care

Without question, the follow-up care of a simple wound is at least as important as the techniques used in its initial repair. The first dressing should be changed within a few days because early inspection gives early clues of incipient or actual infection. The prophylactic use of antibiotics is never justified; antibiotics should be reserved for treatment of actual infection. Simple skin wounds seldom become infected even in the presence of heavy contamination.

The prophylactic use of tetanus antitoxin also can only be condemned. The purpose of tetanus antitoxin is to neutralize the toxin of the *Clostridium* organisms, and the toxin is never present at the time of the original injury. If tetanus invasion seems likely, the wound should be inspected at least every day. When and if evidence of tetanus infection

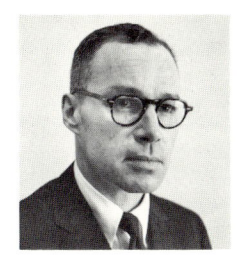

James T. Metzger, M.D.
Delaware Hospital, Wilmington

Doctor Metzger is Attending Plastic Surgeon at Memorial Hospital, Wilmington General Hospital, Delaware Hospital, and several other hospitals in Wilmington, Delaware. He is also Consulting Plastic Surgeon at the U.S. Naval Hospital in Philadelphia and the Alfred I. du Pont Institute of the Nemours Foundation in Wilmington. He is a Fellow of the American College of Surgeons and a member of the Society of Plastic and Reconstructive Surgery.

appears, immediate hospitalization for wound drainage, administration of high-potency broad-spectrum antibiotic therapy, and massive doses of tetanus *human antitoxin* are clearly indicated. Of course, with any wound, a prophylactic immunization of tetanus *toxoid* should be given. This may act as a booster dose in the patient who has been previously actively immunized or, in an unimmunized person, will act as the first of a series of doses leading to active immunity.

Solving the Problem of Emergencies

As far as I am concerned, a simple laceration is always poorly timed. What can be more upsetting than to have a patient rush into a crowded waiting room wrapped in a bloody towel, frantic and frightened? A simple solution to this problem is to have a back room to which the patient can be promptly removed. There you can assess the extent of the injury and, if the wound is simple, reassure the patient and allow him to rest and recover before repair of the wound is begun. If you are fortunate enough to have telephone notification of such a wound from someone qualified to determine its seriousness, a regular appointment at the close of the day's schedule can be arranged. If the wound is indeed simple, speed is seldom essential. A reasonable lag between the time of injury and repair will often result in a quiet and cooperative patient instead of an agitated and unhappy doctor-patient-wound relationship.

Nothing is more distressing — or unnecessary — than a painful procedure, which is usually the result of the patient's fear and the doctor's impatience. The wound should be carefully infiltrated with 1% procaine and 15 drops of injectable Adrenalin® to the ounce. Any wound must also be repaired with the patient in the recumbent rather than the sitting position.

With adequate anesthesia in a field made bloodless by Adrenalin®, the wound can be excised and lightly undermined to produce an adequate sewing edge. The skin can then be approximated with closely placed interrupted sutures of 4-0 or 5-0 atraumatic nylon. If in the course of repair some blood vessels continue to bleed, they can be ligated by transfixion sutures of atraumatic plain 4-0 gut.

Do Away with Archaic Instruments

Chances are, equipment for repairing wounds in the office (and even in the emergency room of some community hospitals) has not been recently reviewed and replaced. If instruments are archaic, cuts and cusses are of equal frequency.

To repair any simple laceration, the following are essential:

1. a #15 Bard-Parker knife blade and #3 handle
2. the finest Adson dura forceps with teeth
3. Stevens tenotomy scissors
4. a fine diamond jaw needle holder
5. a simple skin hook
6. a 5 cc. Luer-Lok syringe
7. a new 24- or 26-gauge needle
8. 4-0 plain atraumatic surgical gut
9. 4-0 atraumatic nylon
10. 5-0 atraumatic nylon
11. 6 mosquito hemostats
12. 4 surgical towels
13. 12 3 x 3 sponges
14. 30 ml. medicine glass
15. 1 metal cup
16. 1 ampule of injectable Adrenalin®
17. gloves
18. aqueous Zephiran®
19. Mayo stand, tray, wrapping, linen, and sterilizing facilities

Just one last word: let us never forget that patients may be patient; often doctors are not. Cuts can be cleanly repaired and the cusses sharply reduced by the proper preparation of a simple laceration set, a quick inspection to determine the involvement of important anatomic structures, arrangement for a quiet and cooperative patient, and repeated follow-up of the wound itself.

QUESTIONS AND ANSWERS

Q. *When should sutures be removed?*

A. That depends on the appearance of the wound. Wound healing is never complete in less than 14 days, and, if sutures are removed before this, steps should be taken to support the edges of the wound during the period of final healing. This is best done by the application of transverse gauze strips cemented by collodion (U.S.P., not flexible) until healing has been attained. It is frequently advisable to leave sutures in place during the entire 14-day period.

Q. *You suggest nylon sutures. Is there a place for other material?*

A. I select nylon as the primary skin suture because of its elasticity. Any wound swells to some degree. Newer fibers which are thixotropic (having "molecular memory" such as polyethylene) expand but then contract. Other suture materials, such as annealed stainless steel wire, silk, or cotton, are basically inelastic and will commonly produce stitch marks as a result of resistance against normal postoperative swelling.

Q. *Do you ever use sedatives before the repair of a simple laceration?*

A. Of course. A frightened patient can always be quieted. The judicious and careful use of morphine can only be recommended. The "hold-and-holler" techniques widely employed have no place in modern therapy.

Q. *You state that tetanus antitoxin is never acceptable. What about possible medicolegal action?*

A. There is abundant evidence in the medical literature that tetanus antitoxin is not only ineffective in the classic 1500-unit dose, but also potentially dangerous. Any litigation on this point can, as of today, be rather easily refuted.

chapter 7

COMPLAINTS ABOUT THE SKIN

THE PLAGUE OF ADOLESCENCE, ACNE

Almost every adolescent has acne, yet our knowledge of its pathogenesis has accumulated slowly. From what we do know, it is fair to assume that the lesions of acne are associated with increased activity of hair follicles and sebaceous glands during adolescence. This increase seems to be touched off by a change in status of sex hormones. We know that acne is exceedingly rare during normal childhood and in people whose skin maintains the characteristics of childhood, either from hormonal lack or from inherited constitution. The texture of these skins can be considerably altered at any age by the administration of androgens, which will increase the growth of hair-and-sebaceous-gland units and produce acne. The degree of acne depends on the amount of hormones given and the susceptibility of the individual.

Hair and sebaceous glands, which form an inseparable unit on most parts of the skin, are the sites of acne lesions. Considering the dense population of these units on the face, it is remarkable that so few of them are affected. One fault leading to acne lesions is the closure of the gland orifice by keratin scales and sebum. In time, sebum and soft lanugo hairs pile up, rupture the follicle wall and spread into the dermis. As irritating foreign materials, they cause inflammation which, if it spreads to neighboring follicles, results in acne that is cystic, indurated, and scarring. Other faults, such as tissue edema and possible chemical alterations in sebum, require further study to determine their relationship to acne.

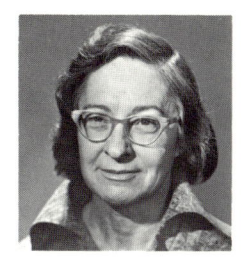

Frances M. Keddie, M.D.
University of California, Los Angeles

Doctor Keddie is an Associate Clinical Professor of Medicine (Dermatology) and a Research Associate in Dermatology at the University of California School of Medicine, Los Angeles. She is a Diplomate of the American Board of Dermatology and Syphilology, and has been President of the San Francisco Dermatology Society and Chairman of the Section on Dermatology of the California Medical Association.

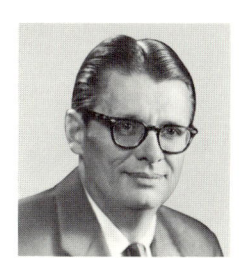

Thomas H. Sternberg, M.D.
University of California, Los Angeles

Doctor Sternberg is an Assistant Dean and a Professor of Medicine (Dermatology) at the University of California School of Medicine, Los Angeles. He is a Diplomate of the American Board of Dermatology and Syphilology; a Fellow of the American Academy of Dermatology and Syphilology; and a member of the American Dermatologic Association.

Steroids and Antibiotics

In treating severe cystic and scarring acnes, which do so much damage to the psyche as well as to the skin, corticosteroids can be safely and successfully used to subdue the inflammation, no matter how severe. When steroids are given in sufficient doses for a long enough period of time, the response is rapid, and once inflammation has subsided, only small doses are necessary to sustain improvement. Failure frequently results when the initial dose is not large enough to cause prompt regression of the already existing lesions. Generally, we use, with good results, a starting daily dose of 16 to 24 mg. of triamcinolone or from 4 to 6 tablets of 0.75 mg. dexamethasone. This initial dosage is continued for one to two weeks. When improvement is satisfactory, a maintenance level is established by gradually decreasing the dose in the usual way. At first we used an antibiotic in conjunction with steroids but later found it unnecessary, except in rare instances. Ordinarily, complete control of this type of acne can be maintained with corticosteroids until such a time as the acne wears itself out and spontaneously disappears.

No conclusion can be drawn about the mode of action of the corticosteroids in acne. It may be that their success is due less to the suppression of the local inflammation than to some regulatory effect on the general hormonal situation. *We have not tried this treatment for juvenile or ordinary pustular acne nor do we advise it.* However, it does provide a method of preventing the severe scarring associated with deep cystic and pustular acne. And in our experience the prolonged use of corticosteroids in young people, with proper medical control, has not been accompanied by any serious side effects.

Antibiotics frequently control inflammation in acne, but the reason they do is not entirely clear. The explanation that microorganisms in the lesions contribute to the inflammation and are inhibited or destroyed by antibiotics may, in part, be true. However, acne lesions are frequently found to be sterile for bacteria. Furthermore, the doses that are effective are usually much lower than those needed to control systemic infections. For example, acne inflammation may be controlled with as little as 125 to 250 mg. of tetracycline daily.

Topical Therapy

In less severe cases the most widely used remedies are cleansing and degreasing agents to relieve the superficial plugs in the follicles. Used alone or with keratolytic agents they prevent, to some extent, the more serious and extensive pustular and cystic lesions from developing.

Today the best of these preparations are combinations of drying and keratolytic agents, with specially prepared sulfur, in a lotion or in a greaseless base. Many are tinted and so act to cover the lesions as well as to treat them. Additional topical therapy with lotions containing antibiotics and steroids are frequently useful to control superficial irritation and infection.

A final note on topical care: telling adolescents not to pick or squeeze lesions is well-meant but seldom-followed advice. Instead they can be told to use a hot compress and gentle pressure to remove excess sebum from some lesions and to use a drying lotion afterward.

Diet, Drugs, and Hormones

Almost all patients suspect that what they eat either causes or contributes to their acne. And generally most practitioners tell their acne patients to eliminate certain foods. Except for chocolate, shellfish, and halogen compounds, food and drugs seem to make little difference in the severity or duration of acne. Certainly the sebaceous glands manufacture the sebum, probably from the glycogen found in abundance within the glands, but they do not act as excretory organs for the fats ingested or circulating in the blood. Vitamins, too, have found favor from time to time in the treatment of acne but their role, if any, in relation to the function of the sebaceous glands is not clearly understood.

The influence of hormones, particularly androgens, on the activity of the pilosebaceous glands and the production of acne has already been mentioned. Yet despite the relationship, treatments to counteract hormone-induced activity of these glands have been tried and found to fail in the majority of cases. In short, there is no reliable form of hormone therapy useful for the prolonged treatment of ordinary acne.

QUESTIONS AND ANSWERS

Q. *Do you use X-ray therapy in acne?*

A. We have not used X-ray for treating acne for many years. There are many opinions about both the benefits and the possible hazards of X-ray therapy. In our opinion, the balance has tipped against X-ray therapy because we think the antibiotics and steroids produce equal or better results with fewer potential hazards.

Q. *You say halogen-containing drugs are detrimental to acne; what about the use of iodized salt?*

A. Because even a trace of iodide or bromide can contribute to or even cause acne lesions, such things as iodized salt and bromide headache remedies should be avoided.

ATOPIC DERMATITIS—
OR WHATEVER YOU CALL IT

Much has been written about atopic dermatitis, but this disorder remains difficult to diagnose and extremely difficult to treat. In fact, there is even some question about what to call it, some preferring "neurodermatitis" or "eczema." No matter what it is called, however, there are certain basic principles in the diagnosis and treatment to keep in mind when a patient complains of a skin rash that does not go away, especially one that itches.

A number of things may be involved in a patient's skin disorder, including — obviously — contactants such as clothing, industrial materials, cosmetics, and household products. A person with a low tolerance for itching may cause secondary infection by scratching, or scratching may cause irritation that causes more scratching in a perpetual vicious cycle. Since the itching is often worse at night, he may make the skin lesions worse without being awake enough to know what he is doing. Some people have a problem of sweat retention, with little itching vesicles that form under the skin and then break and are easily infected when they are scratched. Occasionally a bout of contact dermatitis, such as poison ivy, seems to touch off a recurring atopic dermatitis. Metabolic disturbance may be involved, such as the mildly hypothyroid state in which the patient's skin becomes excessively dry. Many dry-skinned people who are also thin and hyperactive have neurodermatitis, however, so hypothyroidism need not be a factor. Seborrheic dermatitis or psoriasis may co-exist with atopic dermatitis.

Flare-ups appear to coincide with emotional stress. And atopic dermatitis occurs often in people with family histories of allergic conditions. There seems little point, however, in arguing over whether atopic dermatitis is an allergic or psychosomatic disturbance. When someone has a severe outbreak of atopic dermatitis and is hospitalized, there is usually a complete remission, regardless of the type of therapy. Then, when the patient returns home, his dermatitis reappears. Allergists interpret this sequence of events to mean that the patient was allergic to something in his environment. But physicians who emphasize the psychosomatic aspects of illness believe the patient improved because he was removed

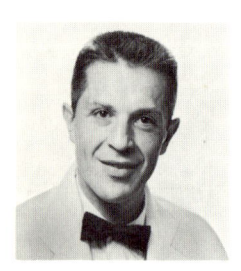

Sidney Olansky, M.D.
Emory University

Doctor Olansky is Professor of Medicine at Emory University School of Medicine, Atlanta, Georgia. He is a past president of the American Venereal Disease Association and a past chairman of the National Serology Advisory Committee of the Surgeon General. Among his professional affiliations are the American Dermatological Association, the American Academy of Dermatology and Syphilology, and the American College of Physicians.

from psychic stresses that triggered his skin eruptions.

There seems little reason to doubt that emotional factors are important, but it seems equally true that they must work on an atopic soil to produce a skin reaction. Patients with less vulnerable skin seem to express their emotional problems with other types of illnesses.

But it does seem that atopic dermatitis, whether preceded or followed by emotional upsets, occurs in patients who have had infantile eczema, hay fever or asthma, or whose relatives have had these disorders. Contrary to usual beliefs, children with atopic dermatitis do not always "outgrow it." Atopic dermatitis often persists into adulthood or reappears then, sometimes with characteristics different from those in childhood. Many of these patients go through life believing that they are allergic to various foods on a basis of skin tests performed during their infancy or later in life, but we have no proof that food allergies cause atopic dermatitis. Although certain foods may produce positive results in scratch tests, they may not produce an allergic reaction when ingested; it is far more likely that contactants (such as wool) and inhalants (such as dust) cause atopic dermatitis.

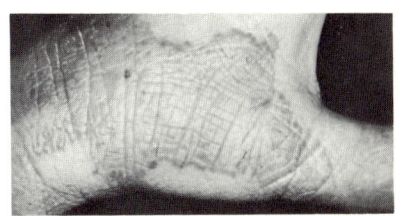

Figure 1 — Chronic eczema; patient had personal and family history of atopy.

Atopic dermatitis typically appears as symmetrically distributed lesions accompanied by chronic thickening of the skin, fine uniform scaling, and exaggerated skin markings. In severe cases, the lesions may cover so much of the body that they are difficult to distinguish from exfoliative dermatitis, but they are usually seen on the flexural areas of the knees and elbows, the face, neck, the backs of the hands and feet, and in skin folds, especially the axillary and inguinal folds (Figure 1).

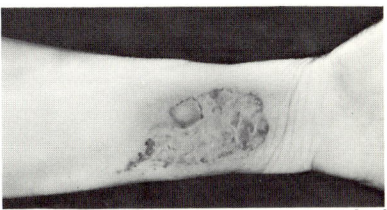

Figure 2 — Chronic eczema; patient had atopic history as child and adult.

Aberrant Forms

There are also aberrant forms of atopic dermatitis. Although some may disagree, I feel that many of the so-called housewife's eczemas or chronic hand eczemas are actually atopic dermatitis (Figure 2). Many of the patients I see have family or personal histories of atopy, and this might well explain the chronicity of their hand eczemas. Nummular eczema, coin-shaped patches of eczema occurring in various sites on the body, may well be another manifestation of atopic dermatitis (Figure 3).

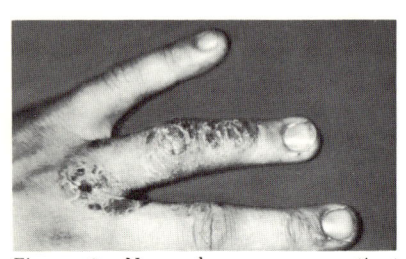

Regardless of the site of its lesions, the course of atopic dermatitis is marked by flare-ups and remissions, and by extreme chronicity. Changes in temperature usually cause a flare-up of the eruption and so may emotional problems. Secondary infection and contact dermatitis are frequently superimposed as a result of scratching and attempts at self-medication with the most easily accessible local remedies.

Figure 3 — Nummular eczema; patient had a strong atopic history in childhood.

History Helps Decide Individual's Treatment

Once you establish that the patient has atopic dermatitis, his history will help you decide what causes the condition and what aggravates it. Because atopic dermatitis is chronic and flares up often, the chances are the patient will have some idea about its cause. He will probably remember that itching is worse — or at least that he scratches more — when he is upset about something. But, more valuable, he may remember that the dermatitis cleared up under certain conditions: perhaps when he was out of doors nearly all day for several days in succession, or when he wore certain kinds of clothing. If certain allergens can be pinpointed, the patient can be desensitized or at least can be warned to avoid the things that produce skin reactions. Some patients may benefit from psychiatric treatment if their skin eruptions seem most strongly related to emotional upsets, but I am inclined to look for more tangible irritants.

Aside from avoiding irritants, patients need symptomatic therapy: sedatives and antipruritics, and topical steroids. Steroids should be used in combination with antibiotics when the latter are warranted by infection. Try to overcome dryness of the skin with oil baths and to prevent the patient from irritating his skin by excessive use of soap and "home cures."

As a last resort, give cortisone or one of its derivatives systemically. But use it sparingly; it is so remarkably effective that patients may become dependent on it. Besides, prolonged use of cortisone or its analogues can produce side effects, which are well known. In other words, the use of cortisone is sometimes justified, such as when the dermatitis becomes incapacitating and is resistant to other therapy, but it is best to reserve its use for these times. Remember, once you place a patient with disseminated neurodermatitis on cortisone therapy, it is almost impossible to obtain successful results with any other modality.

RECURRING CANKER SORES

Some diseases seem to elude medical attention not because of their great rarity, but, instead, because of their great commonness. Such diseases are readily diagnosed by the patient's relatives, friends, and neighbors who usually volunteer that they get the same thing themselves, and, furthermore, that there is nothing much good for it.

This appears to be the case with recurring oral aphthae (a term that goes back to Hippocrates) which are more commonly called canker sores. A recent British survey indicated that 1 in 5 persons in the general population suffer from them at one time or other in their lives. For most people, the sores come infrequently and cause only a minor inconvenience, but for others the disease can be severe, unrelenting, and almost totally disabling.

What Causes Them?

The cause of recurring oral aphthae is unknown. One thing seems certain despite some medical articles and considerable lay prejudice: aphthae are *not* due to the herpes simplex virus. Recurring herpetic fever blisters occur around the mouth, not inside it.

Many patients who suffer from episodic aphthae relate the disease to emotional factors. In women, for example, this disease, like most obscure diseases, is often blamed on either the menstrual flow or its cessation at the menopause. Food allergy to chocolate, walnuts, and so forth, is another commonly blamed offender although it is certainly not responsible for the vast majority of cases. Other dietary and digestive disturbances are also sometimes blamed.

How Prevalent Are They?

The condition is common. It is somewhat more prevalent in women than in men. It often begins in adolescence or early adult life but may occur at any age from childhood on.

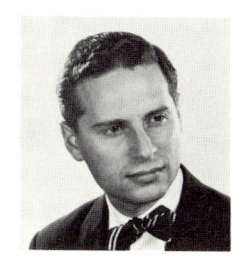

E. William Rosenberg, M.D.
University of Tennessee

Doctor Rosenberg is Assistant Professor of Dermatology at the University of Tennessee and Consultant in Dermatology at the Veterans Administration Hospital and the U.S. Naval Hospital in Memphis. He has been writing since his medical school days when he worked part-time for the International News Service. His professional affiliations include the American Academy of Dermatology and the Society for Investigative Dermatology.

How Easy Are They to Diagnose?

The lesions of recurring aphthous stomatitis occur on the inner aspects of the lips, the buccal mucosa, the tongue, and the gums. They can occur anywhere inside the mouth but are less common on the tonsillar pillars, helping to differentiate them from the lesions of herpangina.

Often the patient will sense an outbreak before it appears, complaining of a peculiar burning or stinging sensation somewhere in the mouth. The lesion begins with a small area of redness. Soon thereafter, the site develops into a superficial slough, about 1 to 3 mm. in size, covered by a white-gray membrane. The extreme amount of pain reported often seems inconsistent with the small size of the lesion. Later, the lesion may enlarge to nearly 1 cm. in diameter and become much deeper. Outbreaks consist of anything from a single small lesion to involvement of almost the entire oral mucosa.

A history of previous attacks and the absence of gross cervical lymphadenopathy help to differentiate aphthosis from the unusual occurrence of primary herpetic stomatitis in an adult. Other conditions with which aphthae may be confused include erosions from ill-fitting dentures, drug eruptions, erythema multiforme, pemphigus, and herpangina. Oral manifestations of pernicious anemia, cyclic neutropenia and the leukemias can be differentiated by blood studies. The nosologic status of conditions like Behcet's syndrome in which aphthous ulcerations are associated with eye and genital involvement is unclear; they may be closely related. In most cases, however, the diagnosis is straightforward and easy.

What Is Their Usual Clinical Course?

There is a wide variation in the amount of trouble caused by aphthae. For most patients the tendency to recurring oral ulcerations is extremely chronic, lasting from 10 to 20 years or more. The majority of patients suffer from only a few small ulcers that occur less than 3 or 4 times a year and heal spontaneously in 1 to 3 weeks. Other patients who suffer similarly infrequent but more severe attacks are subject to a periodic breakdown of large areas of oral and lingual mucosa associated with great pain, inability to eat, and a foul breath. It may well be that much of what is called "trench mouth" is this sort of severe aphthous outbreak, secondarily overrun by the oral flora. Finally there is a small number of unfortunate persons who suffer almost continually from aphthae of greater or less severity. They get a new outbreak every two or three weeks and the lesions no sooner heal than others appear. When they get the severe ulcerative form of the disease, their misery is extreme and nearly constant and may last over many years.

Is There a Standard Treatment?

The list of suggested treatments runs from aureomycin to *Lactobacillus* to trichloroacetic acid to X-ray and is nearly endless. Since aphthae are common, occur at irregular intervals, and are always self-healing, they afford a perfect opportunity for the physician to choose some favorite treatment that he is convinced is effective (but isn't). However, there is some value in those treatments the doctor himself believes in because there is some evidence that the interested, optimistic physician helps, perhaps by suggestion, to shorten and ease attacks.

Repeated smallpox inoculations as a means of preventing attacks is an excellent example of the role that suggestion plays. This treatment is frequently used in the therapy of recurring herpes simplex and came into favor when aphthae were thought to be a manifestation of herpes infection. Since we now know that this is not true, we must assume that any beneficial effects are due to suggestion — which is probably the case in herpes, too.

Is Steroid Therapy Helpful?

Some studies, and my own experience, indicate that the corticosteroids given in adequate doses are highly effective in shortening and aborting an attack. Usually 4 tablets of one of the standard preparations (like prednisone or prednisolone) taken for three to six days will bring satisfactory improvement.

Some patients seem to get by with a lower total dose of steroid if they use one of the topically-active forms of corticosteroid (hydrocortisone is, cortisone is not; prednisolone is, prednisone is not) and suck on the tablet until it dissolves instead of swallowing it. The recently introduced Kenalog® in Orabase® includes the topically-effective triamcinolone acetonide in a special ointment base that will stick to the oral mucosa. It has seemed to be of some limited benefit in a few cases.

The steroids are of most value in patients who get infrequent but severe attacks. They are probably not justified in the sporadic mild attack. In patients with continuing severe attacks, the considerations of extensive, long-term use of steroids are the same as in arthritis and other disorders where their usefulness in alleviating symptoms must be weighed against possible side effects.

Patients with extensive erosions may obtain some symptomatic relief with Xylocaine Viscous Syrup®, especially before attempting to eat. Cold malted milkshakes are useful in supporting patients in too much pain to eat.

BAD DANDRUFF

If we were to rate the importance of medical problems according to the number of over-the-counter products sold for them, then high on the list would be dandruff. This problem has reaped millions of dollars for shampoo manufacturers . . . and for the TV networks, newspapers, and magazines that advertise their products. It is not apt to be so rewarding for you, but it still represents an important part of dermatologic care.

To consider dandruff from a medical viewpoint, we can first think about what it actually is. As you know, the term "dandruff" includes a variety of conditions. However, when the layman refers to it, he is usually thinking of the flaking process which occurs in what we shall call "normal" scaling. The entire scalp may be covered with loose dry scales — a result of the continuous flaking off of the outer layers of the epidermis, not the result of dried-out sebum, as some people think. These gray or white scales accumulate in round patches and, when the head is combed, brushed, or scratched, fall as "snow" onto the shoulders. Sometimes itching accompanies scaling, and the scalp may show a thickened, reddened appearance due to constant scratching; usually, however, it appears dull and gray.

This scaling condition may persist unchanged in a person for his lifetime, or it may worsen only slightly. For many patients, however, complaints of scaliness represent the symptoms of one of several scalp diseases. The commonest of these are: seborrheic dermatitis, psoriasis, and lichen simplex chronicus (circumscribed neurodermatitis). They may occur in varying degrees of severity, and they may occur together. Here is what you can do about them.

Seborrheic Dermatitis — The Most Common Cause

Seborrheic dermatitis, the most common inflammatory scalp disease, may occur in acute, subacute, or chronic forms (Figure 1). It can produce excessive oiliness of the scalp as well as greasy scaling, exudation, crusting, and redness. Yellow-brown, greasy crusts with red margins may occur on the scalp and along the hairline.

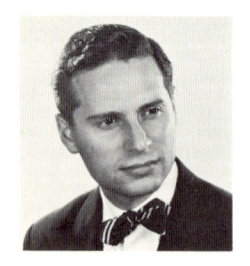

E. William Rosenberg, M.D.
University of Tennessee

Doctor Rosenberg is Assistant Professor of Dermatology at the University of Tennessee and Consultant in Dermatology at the Veterans Administration Hospital and the U.S. Naval Hospital in Memphis. He has been writing since his medical school days when he worked part-time for the International News Service. His professional affiliations include the American Academy of Dermatology and the Society for Investigative Dermatology.

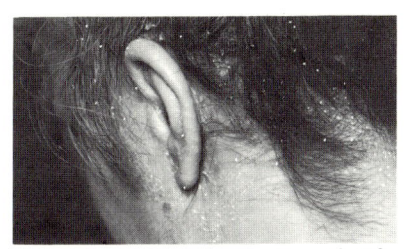

Figure 1—In this common type of seborrheic dermatitis, loose flakes pervade the hair. Scaling along scalp margins and around ear resembles psoriasis.

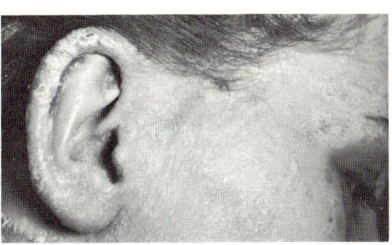

Figure 2—Psoriasis on face and ear has extended into scalp. Typical psoriatic patch may be seen behind the ear.

When excessive oiliness occurs without scaling or flaking and without redness and scaling at the scalp margins, you can usually control it with any good soap or nonsudsing detergent, such as tincture of green soap or Acidolate®. You may have to reassure your patient that he can wash his hair as often as necessary to keep it clean; some people believe, surprisingly, that washing the hair oftener than once a week is dangerous.

When light scaling accompanies excessive oiliness of the scalp, a medicated shampoo is frequently all the patient will need. Prescribe a cleansing preparation such as Fostex Cream® which contains sulfur and salicylic acid, or one which contains tar. Frequently his regular shampoo and an application of Selsun® will do the job.

However, when *heavy* scaling and flaking accompanies oily scalp, you need something more. First, have your patient massage a tar-sulfur-salicylic acid ointment, such as Pragmatar®, thoroughly into the scalp and allow it to remain overnight or, better still, for 24 hours. Then have him wash his hair with tincture of green soap. Have him continue the treatment daily for about three days, then twice a week for two more weeks. If the condition has not cleared after this course of treatment, treat it as though it were psoriasis. The tar-sulfur-salicylic acid ointment also controls redness and scaling at the scalp margins. Some of the newer steroid creams, too, should control it if rubbed in vigorously and frequently. If the patient is still not better, treat him as if he has psoriasis.

Psoriasis — The Most Obstinate

You should strongly suspect psoriasis as a cause of dandruff if you find psoriasis elsewhere on the body, but remember that often it may attack only the scalp.

Psoriasis of the scalp (Figure 2) is often confused with seborrheic dermatitis. In fact, about the only way you can differentiate the two is by the greater severity of psoriasis and its resistance to the usual antiseborrheic preparations. Also, psoriasis is more likely to occur in patches, while seborrheic dermatitis is more likely to involve the entire scalp.

The thick heavy scale of psoriasis often responds to treatment with a mixture of salt and phenol such as Baker's P&S Liquid®. Have the patient rub this into the scalp twice a day for five days, then wash it out. Repeat two or three times until the condition clears. If the psoriasis persists, try one of the synthetic corticosteroid creams along with an occlusive dressing. Have the patient rub the cream into the scalp, cover it with a sheet of plastic such as Saran Wrap®, and secure it by a hairnet or plastic shower cap. The patient should keep it in place overnight and as long as possible during the following day. The treatment should be repeated for 14 to 21 days. If this fails, I suggest you refer him to a specialist who probably is more accustomed (or more resigned) to the obstinacy of psoriasis.

Lichen Simplex Chronicus — The Most Itchy

Cartoonists portray concentration and intellectual effort by the visual cliché of someone scratching the back of his head; they might also portray the effects of lichen simplex (localized neurodermatitis) the same way, for it commonly occurs on the back of the head — and it always itches. Crusted, sharply defined, reddened patches form because of constant scratching to relieve the itch (Figure 3).

This intense itching helps to differentiate lichen simplex from seborrheic dermatitis and psoriasis. Intense itching is not characteristic of either of the two other diseases. Lichen simplex is often obscured by seborrheic dermatitis, which may accompany it, but when the seborrheic dermatitis clears, the lichen simplex remains. For lichen simplex, the new corticosteroid creams (both with and without occlusive dressing) are useful; however, this disease sometimes responds only to intradermal or subcutaneous injection of corticosteroids under the scaly patches.

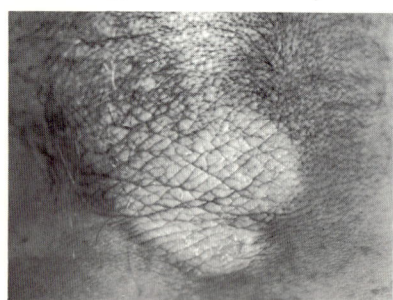

Figure 3—Lichen simplex chronicus appears as a thickened, grilled patch, shown here on the back of the neck.

In summary, remember, you can control the common forms of dandruff successfully if you:
— advise frequent washing for oily scalp.
— prescribe medicated shampoos for lightly scaling seborrheic dermatitis.
— prescribe tar-sulfur-salicylic acid ointment with shampoo for heavily

scaling seborrheic dermatitis.
— use salt and phenol mixture or synthetic corticosteroids with occlusive dressing for resistant psoriasis.
— infiltrate with injectable steroids for lichen simplex.

QUESTIONS AND ANSWERS

Q. *What causes seborrheic dermatitis?*

A. We really do not know. It may involve the sebaceous glands, as the name implies, but some dermatologists believe seborrheic dermatitis has little to do with sebaceous function.

Q. *Does loss of hair occur in dandruff?*

A. No, not in the common forms of dandruff. In a very severe condition, hair loss may occur but only temporarily. As the condition is corrected, hair growth recurs.

Q. *Should I advise my patient to brush his hair during treatment for dandruff?*

A. Brushing has little effect on the clinical course of dandruff one way or another.

Q. *Does diet affect dandruff?*

A. No, not so far as we know. However, it is interesting to note that an eruption similar to seborrheic dermatitis develops in people who are fed a pyridoxine-deficient diet or who are treated with deoxypyridoxine, a metabolic antagonist of the vitamin.

Q. *Does dandruff occur in children?*

A. Chronic dandruff rarely occurs in children beyond early infancy. (Cradle cap in infants may be a form of dandruff.) It begins usually during adolescence and may persist into adulthood.

DRY SKIN

In treating skin conditions, there are few skills more useful than skill in treating "dry skin," for it is one of the most common complaints — particularly during the wintertime. When patients complain of "dry skin," they actually mean *roughness, scaling, redness, chapping,* or sensations of *burning, stinging,* or *itching*. Although these conditions may look different, there is more than a little truth in the way patients lump them together: all of them *do* involve dry skin. Correcting the dryness will usually relieve the symptoms in these cases, and fortunately we have some new techniques for doing this. I will review some of the more effective ones.

Pointers for Diagnosis

Dryness of the skin appears as a symptom in three types of patients. First are patients with no real skin problem other than dryness: those with so-called winter itch, the many with pruritus senilis, and the ones with what advertising copywriters used to call "dishpan hands." These patients need no treatment other than correction of the skin dryness.

The second type have some other accompanying condition, and, in them, dryness is only part of the symptomatology: those with atopic dermatitis, icthyosis, some cases of scaly chronic dermatitis, and the troublesome tendency toward hyperkeratosis of the palms and soles that often afflicts elderly people. Correcting the dryness in this group is helpful but not curative.

Finally, there are some miscellaneous skin conditions that can be alleviated by treating dryness, such as the scaling, reticulated, reddened areas of "sheet dermatitis" that occur on the legs of bedfast patients. And areas of dry skin with erythema and scaling may occur after long exposure to hot air, as when a person stands or sits near a hot-air register or a space heater, such as a car heater (where the shins are usually affected).

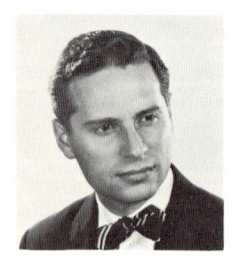

E. William Rosenberg, M.D.
University of Tennessee

Doctor Rosenberg is Assistant Professor of Dermatology at the University of Tennessee and Consultant in Dermatology at the Veterans Administration Hospital and the U.S. Naval Hospital in Memphis. He has been writing since his medical school days when he worked part-time for the International News Service. His professional affiliations include the American Academy of Dermatology and the Society for Investigative Dermatology.

What the Trouble Is

It might seem logical to wet the skin when it is too dry, but experience has shown that bathing always made dry skin worse. Therefore, the traditional advice to these patients has been: "Avoid water. Bathe infrequently." They are told to use cleansing creams and oils instead of soap. The usual treatment is topical greases and creams. In other words, treatment has always been based on the assumption that the skin needed more oil and less water.

In recent years, however, studies have shown that the common feature of all forms of skin dryness is a lack of moisture in the horny outer layers. Oils and skin lipids help prevent dryness chiefly because they help hold water in. The reason that simple washing makes these people worse is that each time they wash, the water rapidly evaporates, taking away the minimal oily matter that has accumulated, leaving the skin drier than ever, and further disorganizing the lamellar scale. There have been a number of studies that have demonstrated this; some of the best have been carried out by Dr. Irvin H. Blank of Harvard Medical School.

Newer Treatment Techniques

Fresh insights into the nature of skin dryness have resulted in radical changes in treatment techniques. Instead of shunning water, your patient with dry skin should soak in it, either by sitting in a tub or by applying wet compresses as often as necessary. He should then dry himself only lightly and, while his skin is still quite damp, apply some greasy ointment that will keep the moisture in. The specific ointment is not important. What *is* important is that the ointment be quite occlusive and that it be applied over damp skin.

The idea of treating dry skin with water plus oil has led to increased use of emulsion bases that contain both oil and water in a stabilized cream. Your patient can apply water and oil simultaneously with one of these products, which are cosmetically acceptable and quite useful for mild cases of dry skin. In severe cases, however, they are seldom as effective as the two-step, soak-then-grease method.

More recently, the idea of treating dry skin with water and oil simultaneously has led to the introduction of several bath oils. These preparations are added directly to a tub full of tap water. All the patient has to do is sit in the water-and-oil emulsion for about 15 minutes and then climb out. He should not use soap, of course, and he should dry himself only lightly. When the correct balance of water and oil is used, the patient's skin will be hydrated and his skin will retain its moisture without feeling greasy. Except for the fact that some patients may dislike climbing out of slippery tubs, and that it may actually be somewhat hazardous for some elderly people (the oils make the tub quite slippery), these oil-bath "treatments" are often used enthusiastically by those who dislike having greases or creams on their skin.

Old-Fashioned Remedy

Our newer knowledge of how oils keep moisture in skin at last provides a scientific rationale for grandma's favorite treatment, rosewater and glycerin. The hygroscopic qualities of glycerin help the skin retain moisture and counteract dryness. For some patients, this old-fashioned remedy works better than any of the newer lotions.

For most patients, the new treatments described will relieve dry skin, whatever its cause. Especially resistant areas may have to be covered with some kind of plastic, such as Saran Wrap®, at least until some progress is made toward controlling the dryness. Remember, though, that relieving the dryness will not of itself "cure" anything. You will also have to diagnose and treat accompanying disorders, if any. And remember, too, that the "dry" scaling that accompanies seborrheic dermatitis is not a true dryness. Patients with seborrheic dermatitis will respond better to more washing and to sulfur and the other standard antiseborrheic measures.

QUESTIONS AND ANSWERS

Q. *What do you recommend as an occlusive ointment to be applied over a limited area of skin immediately after washing, to keep moisture in?*

A. If keeping moisture in is the only consideration, petrolatum still beats all other preparations for real occlusiveness.

Q. *What do you recommend if a patient's skin dryness accompanies a difficult dermatological condition such as atopic dermatitis?*

A. You should treat the skin dryness to give the patient symptomatic relief, but treatment of the atopic dermatitis has to be specific for each patient.

Q. *Is there any particular emulsified cream you would recommend, and any particular bath oil?*

A. There are a number of good preparations. Among the creams I would recommend are Acid Cloak Creme®, Nivea Creme®, Lubriderm® and Lowila Emollient®. Among the better bath oils are Mellobath®, Domol®, Lubath® and Alpha-Keri®.

SKIN RASHES IN THE NEWBORN

Skin rashes are so common in the newborn that it is unusual to find a baby under a week old without one or more skin blemishes. Neonatal rashes usually have no major clinical significance, and they often go unnoticed by the attending physician and the nurses; if they are noticed, they are usually ignored — not recorded, and often not mentioned to the mother.

Unimportant as they may seem to us, skin rashes may be important to mothers of newborn babies. During the baby's first few weeks, they often cause more worry than any other condition. And, they sometimes provoke treatment that is unnecessary and sometimes harmful. We cannot *prevent* many of these rashes but we can and should take the time to discuss them with the mother — to reassure her, tell her how to treat them, and probably most important, when not to treat them at all.

This report describes eight common rashes, and what you can tell the mother about them. The data are based on observation of over 10,000 infants studied in two hospitals over a six-year period.

1. "Diaper Rash"

Rashes in the perianal and gluteal areas — skin areas that have direct contact with feces — occur in about one-third of infants during their first week of life. Generally they are mild with erythema and occasional papules (see Figure 1), but occasionally they are severe, with ulceration and hemorrhages (see Figure 2). We do not know exactly what causes diaper rash in the newborn, but since most diaper rashes develop in the perianal region and do not spread beyond it, the most likely cause seems to be irritation by feces. The newborn infant may be more susceptible to irritation from contact with feces because of his rather fragile, unseasoned skin.

Obviously, the best way to prevent neonatal "diaper dermatosis" is to remove soiled diapers promptly to avoid prolonged contact with feces and resulting maceration. If babies were always changed promptly, diaper rashes might well be rare. Unfortunately, in the hospital, frequent

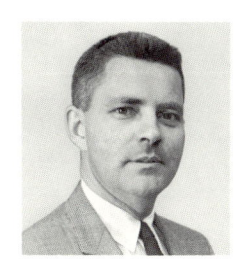

Hans G. Keitel, M.D.
Jefferson Medical College

Doctor Keitel is Professor and Head of the Department of Pediatrics at Jefferson Medical College of Philadelphia, and is associated with three Philadelphia Hospitals: Jefferson, Episcopal, and Philadelphia General. He has served as Instructor in Pediatrics at New York University; as Clinical Assistant and Research Fellow in Pediatrics at Harvard Medical School; and as Assistant Clinical Professor of Pediatrics at Georgetown University.

changing is not always possible during peak nursery loads; at such times, however, it may be helpful to keep the babies lying prone. Babies who lie prone have a lower incidence of diaper rash than those who lie supine. However, while the prone position reduces the incidence of gluteal rash, it increases the incidence of rashes (sheet burns) on the knees and nose.

What about topical medications to *prevent* diaper rash? Our own experience with these has been disappointing. In controlled studies with such medications, we have found that those which contain either antibiotics or a high concentration of silicone sometimes *increase* the incidence of diaper rash. The best measures for preventing and treating gluteal diaper rash are the simple and obvious ones — cleanliness, frequent changes and keeping the baby in the prone position.

It is especially important to discuss the presence of diaper rash with the mother whose infant is about to leave the nursery. Although this tends to be an embarrassing subject and allows the mother to comment on the "inadequacy" of nursing care, a positive approach to the problem is worth trying. You can point out that the baby's skin is extremely sensitive at this age and that even a short period of contact with feces may be irritating. If you initiate the discussion and tell the mother how to cope with diaper rash at home, she is less likely to complain about a nursery failure.

2. "Dry Skin"

Another very common skin condition in the newborn results from dermal flakiness — particularly in lean, "postmature"-looking babies (see Figure 3). In extreme cases the baby looks as if he might have congenital ichthyosis; he may have deep linear grooves — sometimes with evidence of hemorrhage — along the skin lines, particularly in the inguinal, ankle, and wrist areas. There is a natural tendency for nurses and mothers to treat such lesions with ointments and creams. However, we have found that oily medications are not particularly helpful and may predispose the infant to another skin disease, pyoderma. Besides, the dryness will disappear within a week or two whether medications are used or not. This is another condition you should discuss with the mother. By assuring her that it is self-limiting, you will relieve her anxiety and, at the same time, prevent her from overmedicating the infant.

3. Maculopapular Rashes

These are present in almost half of all newborn infants. In severe cases, they look very much like rubella (see Figure 4), except that they are generally somewhat more pronounced on the trunk than on the face.

The neonatal maculopapular rash appears most commonly on the second day of life, starts to fade by the third day, and often disappears by the fifth or sixth day.

The etiology of these rashes is unknown. They do not seem to be due to any particular medication the mother might have received, nor to medications applied to the baby's skin. Treatment is unnecessary. However, mothers tend to worry about them — to feel anxious that something is wrong with the baby, or that they may have done something that caused them. They are relieved to hear that these rashes are present in one-half or more of all newborn babies, that they disappear spontaneously and have no long-term significance.

4. Milia

These are innumerable, minute, whitish yellow papular vesicles commonly found on the nose, forehead, and face and less commonly on the trunk and elsewhere. They are not important unless they are very large "macro-milia" and therefore very noticeable (see Figure 5). If you find "macro-milia" immediately after birth and if erythema is not present, you can be reasonably certain that they are not a sign of pyoderma. Occasionally you will find "macro-milia" that are surrounded by a narrow area of erythema; such lesions have been referred to as "benign pustules." You need not mention the presence of milia unless they are very noticeable, in which case you should tell the mother that they will disappear within a few weeks and that treatment is unnecessary.

5. Periumbilical Erythema

A narrow area of erythema around the umbilical stump is common. If this area is no more than 1 to 2 mm. wide, and if there is no edema or streaking beyond the erythema, you can ignore it (see Figure 6). However, be suspicious of a wider area of erythema, particularly if it is associated with constitutional signs (diarrhea, fever, jaundice); these may indicate cord infection. If you suspect omphalitis, take appropriate cultures and begin antibiotic treatment *immediately*. In this situation, treatment should not wait for a positive bacteriologic diagnosis.

Lately, the incidence of periumbilical erythema has decreased, thanks to the rubber-tubing technique of cord ligation. When metal clamps and linen ties were used for ligation — and particularly if a long length of cord was left — periumbilical erythema was much more common. Then, it was difficult to know whether the erythema was caused by tension on the cord by the weight of the clamp, or whether an active infection was present. The use of rubber tubing for cord ligation is an important advance in neonatal care.

146   complaints about the skin

EIGHT COMMON NEONATAL DERMATOSES

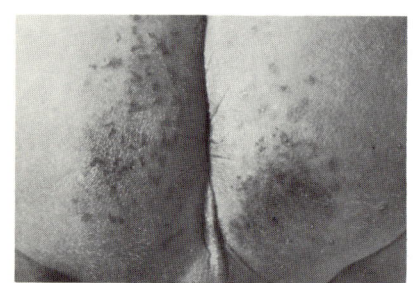

1. Diaper dermatosis

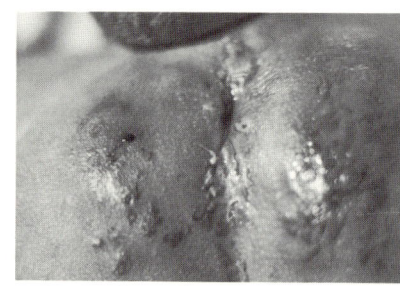

2. Severe diaper dermatosis

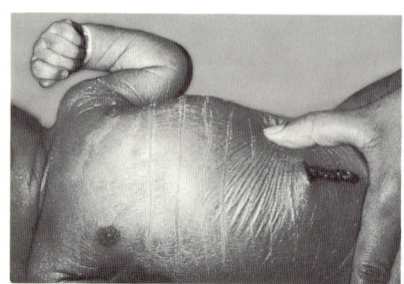

3. Ichthyotic dry skin

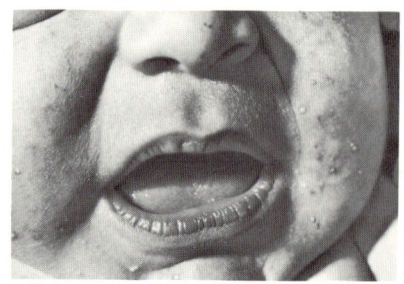

4. Maculopapular rash

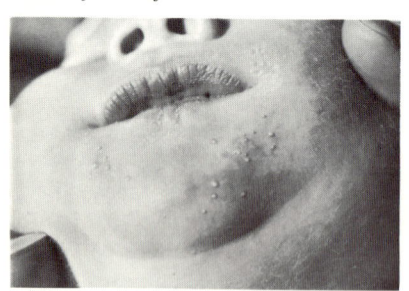

5. Milia

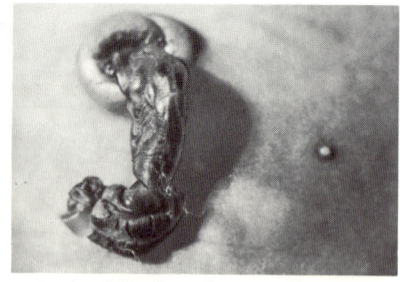

6. Periumbilical erythema with pustule

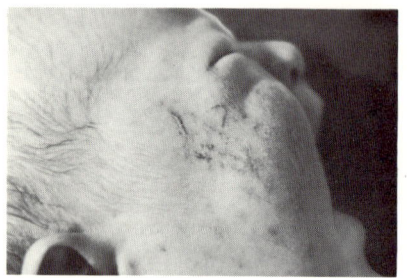

7. Self-inflicted excoriations

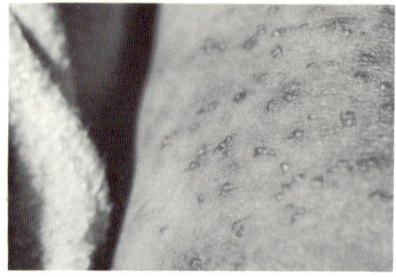

8. Toxic erythema

6. Pustules

Pustules due to staphylococci or streptococci are usually surrounded by erythema. The most common location for pustules is in intertriginous areas such as in the axilla, groin, neck, and behind the ears. When a long length of umbilical cord is left, pustules are quite frequently found under the cord or near the umbilicus close to the necrotic cord (see Figure 6). We now recommend that as little cord be left as possible and that the rubber tubing used for cord ligation completely cover the umbilical stump except for the distal end and a small portion of the proximal stump.

Some nurses treat pustules by wiping them away with 70% alcohol, and they frequently do this without notifying the attending physician a pustule had been present. Although such treatment is ample in most instances, babies with pustules are a threat to the nursery and should be isolated, possibly with their mothers. A smear and culture should be obtained. Some physicians use antimicrobial soaps for preventing staphylococcal nursery infections, but evidence that such soaps are really useful is scarce.

7. Self-Inflicted Excoriations

Almost one-half of newborn babies have facial scratch marks and punctate abrasions which are self-inflicted (see Figure 7). This usually happens just before feeding time when the baby claws at his face. Fortunately, these scratches rarely become infected. I can remember only two infants out of many thousands with self-inflicted scratches who developed infections. Nevertheless, these scratches should be prevented because they are potential portals for infection and they certainly are unattractive. Fortunately, prevention is easily achieved by keeping the nails closely trimmed. Advise the mother to obtain a new nail file and trim the nails down as far as possible. Experienced mothers can trim the baby's nails with scissors but some mothers are fearful of using scissors this way and generally manage better with a file.

8. Toxic Erythema

This dramatic lesion looks like a fleabite, with a papule or vesicle surrounded by a wide area of erythema (see Figure 8). It is benign but often becomes pustular and is accompanied rather commonly by a maculopapular rash. Toxic erythema commonly occurs during the first to fifth day of life and only infrequently thereafter. Treatment is unnecessary. Some investigators believe it is related to allergy (atopy), but we have not been able to confirm this.

chapter 8

COMPLAINTS ABOUT THE FEET

TROUBLESOME ATHLETE'S FOOT

Just because the patient asks, "What's good for athlete's foot," doesn't mean that athlete's foot is what he has. If we accept his casual question as a diagnosis, we are likely to reach for the nearest antifungal agent and thereby do more harm than good.

While it is true that fungus infection of the feet is the more common cause of dry, itchy, hyperkeratotic fissured toewebs, it is not the only cause. What the patient diagnoses as fungus infection may actually be psoriasis, secondary syphilis, bacterial infection, soft corns, cellulitis, or any one of a number of infections that, to him, look and feel like athlete's foot. Antifungal drugs are useless and sometimes harmful in these diseases.

Tight Shoes, Sweat, and Rubber Cement

In addition, the following conditions are often mistaken for athlete's foot:

Maceration — Wearing tight shoes of impervious material, especially in hot weather, causes maceration of the feet. Treatment with antifungal ointments or powders aggravates this condition.

Contact dermatitis — Rubber cement in shoes and dyes in shoes or stockings are the most common causes of contact dermatitis of the feet, which is often mistaken for and treated as athlete's foot (Figure 1). As a help in diagnosing, remember that contact dermatitis more commonly affects the dorsum of toes and feet and the pressure points of the sole, whereas fungal infection is likely to affect the poorly ventilated creases and toewebs. However, this does not mean that every inflammation of the creases and toewebs is caused by fungus; some are caused by bacteria.

Erythrasma — Until recently considered a fungus infection, erythrasma has been shown to be a bacterial infection that may involve the feet as well as the crotch and the armpits. It responds promptly to broad-spectrum antibiotics but is completely resistant to antifungals.

"Athlete's foot of the hands" — Eczematous eruptions of the hands

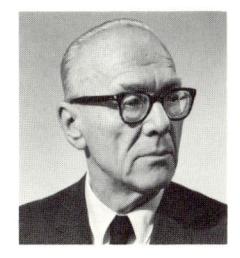

Emory Ladany, M.D.
New York University

Doctor Ladany is Associate Professor of Clinical Dermatology at New York University College of Medicine. He is also Attending Dermatologist at the Veterans Administration Hospital in New York. His affiliations include the American Academy of Dermatology and Syphilology, the International Society of Tropical Dermatology, the New York Academy of Medicine, and the Society for Investigative Dermatology.

152   complaints about the feet

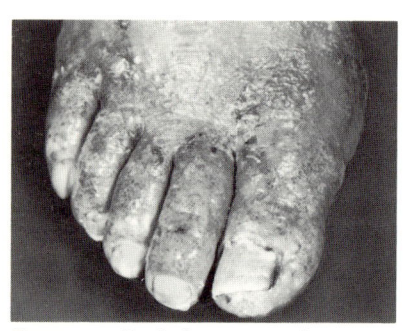

Figure 1 — Typical contact dermatitis, caused by rubber cement in shoes; misdiagnosed and treated as athlete's foot for several weeks.

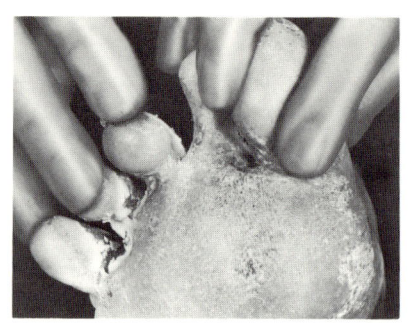

Figure 2—Athlete's foot. Denuded, macerated interspaces were aggravated by strong keratolytic ointments used during the acute infection.

are often mistreated with antifungals. Actually, primary fungus infection of the hands is extremely rare, but if a culture from skin scrapings indicates that it is indeed a fungus infection, it will almost always be the resistant *Trichophyton rubrum* that is responsible. This infection is likely to be found also on the patient's feet, crotch, and many other areas of the body.

The Acute "Fungus" Infection

I never use topical antifungal ointments or powders on any acute skin infection. Any acute flare-up in a chronic fungal infection is almost always caused by bacterial contamination, which is only aggravated by antifungal drugs (Figure 2). Therefore, have the patient apply cold compresses, instead, to relieve the itching and inflammation. If the bacterial infection is purulent, have him use hot soaks and a 2% aqueous solution of gentian violet at first. You may recommend an antibiotic cream or powder — unless the skin is denuded, blistered, and oozing; when it is, limit local treatment to soaks and cool compresses of Burow's solution or potassium permanganate solution. (If lymphangitis or lymphadenitis occur, you may need systemic broad-spectrum antibiotics also.) Only after the oozing and purulent secondary infection have subsided should you treat the underlying fungal infection.

Try Simple Remedies First

The frantic search for an all-powerful single remedy for fungal infection is a mistake. Actually, a clean, dry, well-ventilated foot can be cleared of an occasional fungus infection by a few drops of lemon juice. For chronic athlete's foot, I prefer the simple anti-acne sulfur-resorcin or the salicylic acid cosmetic lotions for daytime application; they are pleasant and effective. They are keratolytic, bacteriostatic and fungistatic, and stay on the feet for many hours without losing their effectiveness. If you wish, prescribe a cream or ointment form of these preparations for application at night. To relieve itching, prescribe lotions and creams with added hydrocortisone or 10-minute applications of cool compresses.

What About Griseofulvin?

Simple fungus infections of the feet can usually be controlled without griseofulvin. Even *Tinea cruris* responds well to local treatment. You should, in fact, use griseofulvin only in very resistant fungal infections, especially those that infect the toenails. If you do use it, be sure to continue the treatment, along with local measures, for from 6 to 10 months, the time needed for complete regrowth of the nail.

In *Trichophyton rubrum* infections, administer griseofulvin along with local applications of ointments and lotions even if there is no nail involvement. Never begin griseofulvin treatment until you have determined what kind of fungus you are dealing with by culture of skin scrapings, because griseofulvin is ineffective, even hazardous, in some fungal infections. For example: although griseofulvin is consistently effective in *Tinea capitis,* it is entirely ineffective in infections caused by monilia (*Candida albicans*), the organisms often found in oozing toe infections, discharging swelling of fingernail tissue, and infections of the webs of the fingers. In these monilial infections, soaks and compresses, nystatin powder, iodochlorhydroxyquin cream, and gentian violet solution are most effective.

Emphasize Prevention

Naturally, the best thing would be to prevent athlete's foot in your patients. But how? Eliminating fungi from their environment is almost impossible; pathogenic fungi occur on apartment floors, bathroom floors, in footwear, on healthy peoples' feet. However, proper foot hygiene can increase resistance to these fungi, so try to impress these rules upon your patients:
• Keep your feet well-ventilated, and dry. Sandals, perforated shoes, even bare feet are preferable to tight hot shoes, especially in hot weather.
• Change socks several times a day if your feet tend to become soggy.
   Your answer to that casual, "Say, Doctor, what's good for athlete's foot?" should be, "Dry, well-ventilated feet — first and foremost."

NEEDLESS FOOT PROBLEMS IN WOMEN

Women's fashions are occasionally ridiculous, but can usually be shrugged off as harmless — with one exception. Fashionable shoes are physically harmful, as every physician who is interested in disorders of the foot knows. How can a male physician begin to understand the mass masochism that makes women cling so tenaciously to footwear that seems to have been designed to cripple them? An interesting and worthwhile question, but not the topic of this article. This article will discuss the orthopedic aspects of women's foot problems and leave the probing of women's psyche to braver souls.

I do not mean to imply that all foot disorders are caused by high-heeled shoes. Other common causes are ill-fitting shoes, obesity, occupations requiring prolonged standing (particularly on unyielding floors), and defects that are either congenital or the result of injury. Naturally, all these causes affect men as well as women. Yet when a colleague recently asked me how many men's feet I had operated on in the past year, I had difficulty remembering a single case; however, in the same period, I operated on dozens of women's feet. My point is that, although both sexes have foot problems, women have more than their share.

Obviously, prevention should be easy, but also obviously, persuading a woman to resist the demands of fashion is impossible or nearly so. So I have learned to compromise. Assisted by pictures and charts, I scientifically explain to my footsore patients the crippling action of high-heeled shoes.

I begin by describing the normal stride: weight first falls on the heel, then shifts forward along the lateral transverse arch first to the fifth metatarsal head (Figure 1). The foot pronates slightly; the weight on the metatarsal area shifts (Figure 2) so that two-sixths rests on the first metatarsus and one-sixth on each of the other four (2-1-1-1). The heel bears a substantial portion of the weight until the moment it lifts from the ground and the big toe pushes off to give a spring to the step.

Compare this normal stride with that of a woman wearing 3″ or 4″ heels. The heel of the fashionably shod woman bears a much smaller share of the weight. The weight is directed forcefully down the in-

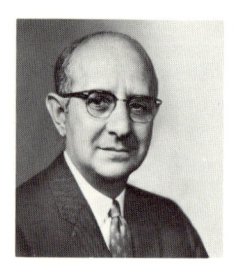

Carlo Scuderi, M.D.
University of Illinois

Doctor Scuderi is Associate Professor of Orthopedic Surgery at the University of Illinois College of Medicine. He also serves as Senior Attending Orthopedic Surgeon at Cook County Hospital and Alexian Brothers Hospital, and as Chairman of the Department of Orthopedic Surgery at St. Elizabeth's and Columbus hospitals, all in Chicago. His professional affiliations include the American Orthopedic Association and the Clinical Orthopedic Society.

clined plane to the metatarsal area (Figure 3). To make matters worse, the toes are jammed forward into a triangular area too small to allow the toes to rest side-by-side (Figure 4). The large toe is angulated laterally, applying abnormal pressure over the metatarsal phalangeal area; eventually the pressure is likely to produce a bunion. The ability of the angulated large toe to push off at the end of each stride is also impaired. The second toe may overlap one of the adjacent toes. The fifth toe may overlap the fourth, applying considerable pressure over the base of the fifth metatarsal and the dorsal surface of the toe (finally producing calluses and corns). The overlapping of toes interferes with the normal 2-1-1-1-1 weight distribution.

Impressive as these diagrams and scientific descriptions are, there is a limit to what science can do. Convincing women to abandon spike heels exceeds that limit. So, next, I admit that high-heeled shoes must be worn at social gatherings (though I secretly wonder why); then having compromised with my conscience to this extent, I tell my patient as firmly as I can that at all other times she must wear low-heeled, broad-toed shoes. I make no claims that this wishy-washy stand is effective; for me, it is more effective than taking an uncompromising stand, no matter how medically defensible that stand may be.

Many of the consequences of failure to wear proper shoes require surgical repair. Because women's vanity is nearly universal, ortho-

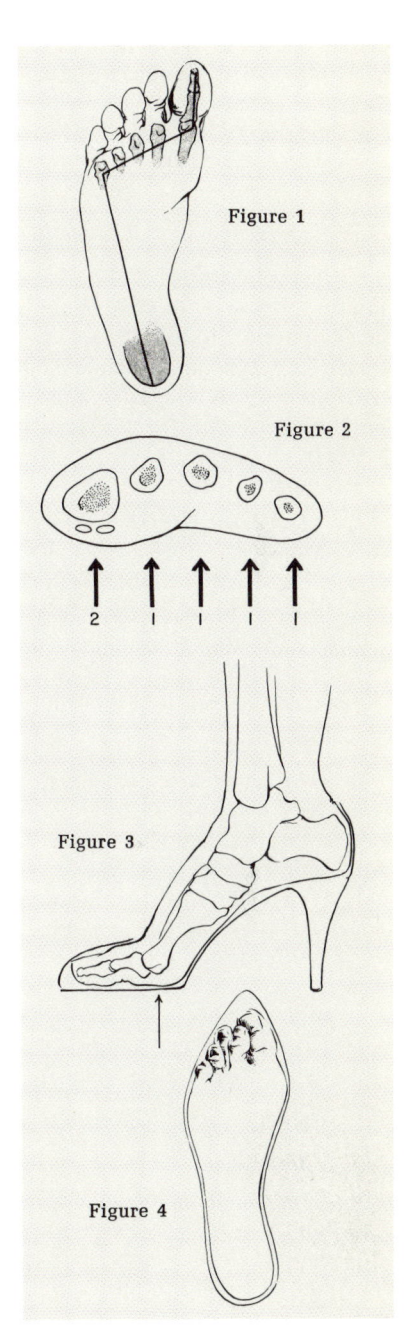

Figure 1

Figure 2

Figure 3

Figure 4

pedic surgeons everywhere find it easy to keep in practice, so you have probably had no trouble finding one to whom you can refer your patients. There are, however, many deformities that can be corrected without surgery, and it is some of these that I would like to discuss.

Fallen Arches

The first rule for management of fallen arches is leave them alone if they are not painful. If they are painful, pads can often relieve the discomfort. I prescribe sponge rubber and leather pads (manufactured by the Kleistone Rubber Company) built up just far enough to relieve discomfort. If the patient's shoes tend to break down, as often happens with obese patients, special shoes with a rigid shank should be prescribed. Of course, you should also advise weight reduction for obese patients.

But most helpful of all, especially in young people with fallen arches, is *nightly* use of special exercises. I especially recommend three to my patients:

(1) "Repeat this three-count exercise 25 times: rise on your toes, then come down on the lateral aspect of the foot with the toes curled, and return to the normal standing position."

(2) "Walk the length of the bedroom 15 times on the lateral aspect of the soles with your toes curled in."

(3) "Practice picking up marbles or pencils with your toes."

If the heel is in calcaneovalgus position, the patient may get some relief from wearing a Thomas heel — that is, a heel which extends about ½" farther toward the toe on the medial side than on the lateral side. Adding a ⅛" or 3⁄16" wedge on the medial side of the heel will also help to shift the heel to a more normal position.

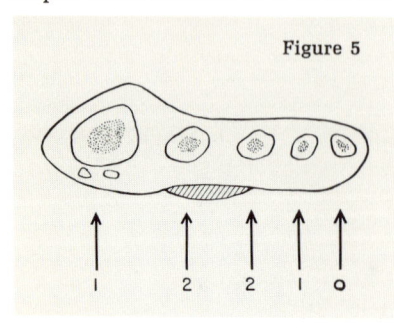

Figure 5

A fallen transverse arch is the result of abnormal weight distribution over the metatarsals. The point of excess weight is usually easily identified because a callus develops there (Figure 5).

After removal of the callus, treatment consists of use of an exactly positioned pad. Measure the distance from the heel to the rear of the callus, then measure the same distance inside the shoe, and place a thin, small metatarsal pad there. The pad will feel strange to the patient at first, but she will get used to it within a week or so. If it does not relieve the symptoms after 10 days, insert a larger pad. Progressively increase both in area and thickness until the most comfortable size is found. The pad ought to be attached permanently in each of the patient's shoes once the proper position and size have been determined.

Other Painful Disorders

A painful heel is a common complaint, which, surprisingly, is not usually caused by a calcaneal spur. Although a spur must sometimes be removed surgically, removal should be attempted only after conservative treatment has failed. Probably a more common cause of painful heel is bursitis over the os calcis. In either case, treatment is the same: padding. If a spur is present, padding will reduce pressure on it until a thick fibrous mass has formed around it and the pain is relieved. This can often be done by inserting heel pads with a round hole at the point of greatest pain. It may take some experimentation to find the most comfortable shape and position of the pad. Also it sometimes helps to have the patient wear heels of different heights on alternate days so that the weight on the heel is never quite the same. Nightly foot soaks in hot Epsom salts and water and application of analgesic balm may help. Also I prescribe oral salicylates for patients with bursitis.

Corns and Calluses

For removing corns and calluses, I suggest 10% salicylic acid in flexible collodion applied each night. I have the patient soak the foot for 15 minutes in hot water the following night, and remove any loose tissue. Repeat the treatment each night until the callus has been removed. If the callus is thick, you can speed treatment by cutting it away with a cuticle cutter or sharp knife. Although removal of corns and calluses is not difficult, the cause (usually ill-fitting shoes) must be eliminated if the patient is to experience lasting relief.

Improperly fitted shoes are frequent causes of sore feet for both men and women, so you ought to have a device for measuring foot size if you treat many patients with foot problems. The one I use is called a Brannock Device. Women are quite likely to prefer shoes that are too narrow, and often seem to be willing to put up with corns that are sure to develop at the pressure points. Still, we ought to do what we can to encourage them to buy wider shoes. One other hint for proper shoe-fitting is this: over-all length and width of the foot are not as important as the distance from the heel to the ball. If this dimension calls for a different shoe size than the over-all length (as it will in the patient who has abnormally long or short toes), it is the ball-heel dimension that should determine the shoe size.

INGROWN TOENAIL

There is an odd circumstance in the treatment of ingrown toenail that frequently changes it from a minor problem to a major one: it is a condition that is easy to relieve but hard to cure. Many techniques for treating the ingrown toenail give only temporary relief because they deal with the toenail rather than the flesh around it. "Ingrown toenail" implies that the disorder is the result of faulty toenail growth, but on the contrary, the nail is ordinarily normal and healthy. If lexicographers had named it "nail-corner-cut-short; flesh-pushed-up," we would not be stuck with an awkward name, but perhaps our treatment would be more precisely directed.

Toenails Should Be Square

Ingrown toenail is most common in the large toe, because it has more soft tissue and bears more weight and more shoe pressure than a smaller toe. It occurs when the patient tries to make his toenails look like fingernails by enthusiastically trimming them to form artistic curves. Taking out the corner of the nail leaves a space, which is filled with soft tissue pushed up by the weight borne by the toe and crowded in by the surrounding shoe or the adjacent toe. When the growing toenail exerts painful pressure on the raised tissue, an ulcer forms. Inflammation and sometimes infection follow. The tissue becomes hypertrophied, hyperplastic, and fibrotic. To relieve the pain, the patient often cuts back the nail still more; this helps, but only until the growing nail again presses against the swollen tissue.

Most surgical procedures for ingrowing toenail are simply more radical versions of the patient's own nail-trimming efforts. The nail may be either partially or completely removed (Figure 1). The important disadvantage of these procedures is the high frequency of recurrence.

The wedge resection (Figure 2) attempts to correct the real problem by removing not the nail but the excess tissue. A lateral wedge of tissue is excised, and the wound is closed with sutures drawn tight to pull the swollen tissue away from the nail. The disadvantages: approximation

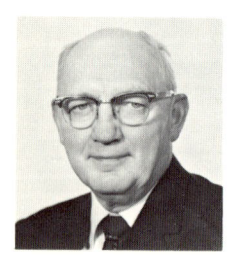

Felix Jansey, M.D.
Northwestern University

Doctor Jansey is an Associate in the Department of Surgery at Northwestern University Medical School and Professor of Surgery at Cook County Graduate School of Medicine. He is also Senior Attending Surgeon at Chicago Wesley Memorial Hospital and Attending Orthopedist at Cook County Hospital and Hines V.A. Hospital. He is a Diplomate of the American Board of Surgery and a Fellow of the International College of Surgeons.

may be difficult because fibrotic tissue is unyielding, and the sutures tend to pull through. Moreover, the offending fibrotic tissue remains.

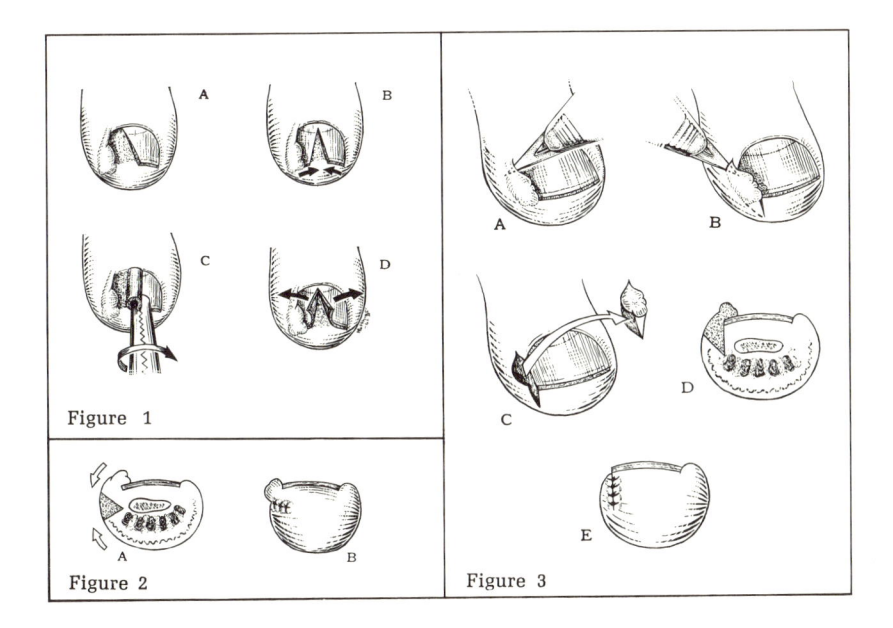

Figure 1

Figure 2

Figure 3

In my experience, these procedures are unsatisfactory because they are often followed by prolonged disability, recurrence is frequent, and the result unsightly. In my operation, the hypertrophied nail fold rather than the nail is removed. As shown in Figure 3, the operation consists of two incisions, one straight and one curved, to form a D- or P-shaped wedge. Slip the scalpel blade between the nail and the overhanging tissue (A). Then make a deep (about ½″), straight incision following the nail margin and extending through the distal tip.

Begin the second incision at the proximal end of the first incision. As you draw the scalpel toward the distal tip (B), tilt the scalpel so that the incision curves away from the nail to encompass all the swollen tissue. Throughout the cut, the imbedded scalpel point remains within the first incision so that, when the second incision joins the first at the distal tip, the wedge of tissue can be lifted free (C). All the fibrosis, ulcer, and granuloma should be excised in one wedge. The scalpel strokes should be continuous to minimize trauma and leave smooth surfaces.

The lateral flap then may be approximated using a mattress suture. However, I find that this is seldom necessary. An encircling strip of adhesive, with a small glob of petrolatum or glycerine on it to prevent sticking, will usually suffice to hold the flap in place. Notice that removal of the wedge of tissue leaves the toe smaller (E); no fold of marginal tissue now projects over the nail. In this respect, the toe now resembles the finger, where little tissue protrudes over the nail — and, incidentally, where ingrown nails are rare.

In the 25 years since I conceived this simple operation, it has served me well; only minimal complications have ever risen. Healing is rapid and permanent because there is no tissue for the nail to grow into.

QUESTIONS AND ANSWERS

Q. *What anesthetic is used?*

A. If your patient is apprehensive, you will probably want to use a general anesthetic; usually, however, local anesthetic is adequate. First, place a small rubber tube about the toe as a tourniquet to minimize oozing, which might obscure vision. Then inject 2 to 4 cc. of procaine into each side of the first metatarsus deep enough to reach the digital nerves. Add a few cc. subcutaneously, but never inject the anesthetic directly into the thickened tissue, for this is painful and ineffective and may spread infection.

Q. *Are any of the nonsurgical treatments effective?*

A. Soaks, ointments, topical anesthetics give only temporary relief. Placing a tuft of cotton under the nail might succeed if the patient does it until the nail has grown beyond the lateral fold; unfortunately such persistence is rare. The cotton does not relieve the pain completely, so the patient usually resorts to cutting back the nail corner again. Temporary relief results, but final cure is delayed.

Q. *Can't recurrence be prevented by permanent removal of the nail?*

A. Yes. It requires excision of the nail matrix and the adjacent layers of the stratum germinativum and stratum corneum in the zone of transformation. Because the zone of transformation lacks a distinctive appearance or a separable cleavage plane, excision may be inadequate, and a deformed nail may regenerate. Obviously, some patients may object to permanent ablation of the nail. Who wants a toe with no nail or only part of one, or a deformed one?

chapter 9

COMPLAINTS PECULIAR TO WOMEN

SIGNS THAT POINT TO BENIGN CERVICAL EROSION

Benign cervical erosion, one of the commonest gynecologic findings, continues to confuse clinicians and mystify investigators. For one thing, it resembles early carcinoma. For another, its nature and cause have been obscured by semantic wanderings and vague concepts. The term, "congenital erosion," is an example: it is not necessarily present at birth, as the term "congenital" implies; nor is there usually a loss of surface epithelium, as the term "erosion" implies (see Figures 1 and 2). Adding to the confusion is the variety of terms to denote essentially the same type of lesion: cervicitis, endocervicitis, eversion, extropion, pseudoerosion, "diseased cervix," heteroplastic endocervical tissue, vermilion halo, and mucoepithelial hyperplasia.

Nor is there any consistency in the theories explaining the cause of cervical erosions. Hormonal changes, variations in pH, infection, irritating secretions of the cervical glands, and, most recently, volume changes of the cervix have been implicated.

The presence of a cervical erosion may be suggested by bleeding (when its fragile surface is injured by coitus or douching) and leukorrhea; more often, however, erosions are asymptomatic and are not suspected until a pelvic examination is performed for some unrelated reason. Even so, the discovery of cervical erosion always poses a vital question:

Is the Lesion Malignant?

You should suspect malignancy if the erosion is irregular and friable, if it seems to be a true ulceration, if it is apparently enlarging, if it is located discretely away from the os, or if it recurs after cauterization. An erosion in a post-menopausal woman is especially alarming when the rest of the organs are atrophic.

A Papanicolaou smear should be obtained in every case of cervical erosion, including young women (even though cervical carcinoma is rare in the teens and twenties). Any erosion that is suspicious in any way should also be biopsied. Admittedly, this policy produces many

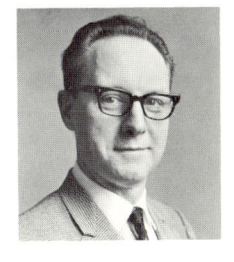

Warren R. Lang, M.D.
Jefferson Medical College

Doctor Lang is a Professor of Obstetrics and Gynecology at Jefferson Medical College of Philadelphia. He is also Associate Director of Obstetrics, and Chief of the Vaginitis Clinic, at Jefferson Medical College Hospital. He has served as chairman of several conferences of the New York Academy of Sciences, and as editor of the transactions of the Inter-Society Cytology Council. He is Secretary-Treasurer of the American Society of Cytology.

164 complaints peculiar to women

| CONGENITAL EROSION | ACQUIRED EROSION |

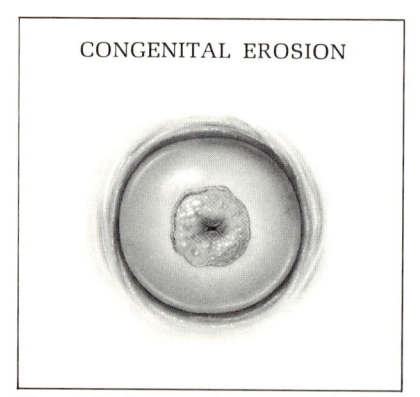

Figure 1—Congenital erosion. Cervical erosions are not true erosions, but rather consist essentially of columnar glandular epithelium on the portio.

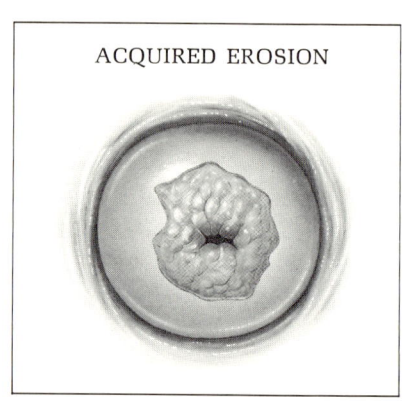

Figure 2—Acquired erosion. Sometimes nabothian cysts (not shown) appear around the area of an acquired erosion when squamous epithelium, advancing toward the anatomical external cervical os, blocks the cervical glands.

negative smears and biopsies and many pathology reports no more revealing or disturbing than "chronic cervicitis," "cystic cervicitis," or "epidermidization," yet it is the only safe policy to follow.

Tips on Diagnosis

Although space does not permit full discussion of the preparation and interpretation of Papanicolaou smears, I would like to point out that I prefer to obtain separate cytologic samples from three sites: the posterior fornix pool (by aspiration), the portio (by scraping), and the endocervix (by aspiration).

There is a choice of several biopsy procedures. Two simple office procedures are spot biopsy, which may miss the carcinoma, and multiple biopsies, which has a better statistical chance of finding it. The coning (ring or annular) biopsy is usually a hospital procedure; though less easily performed, it combines more certain diagnosis and good therapy since it removes the entire area of erosion. If there is any question whatsoever of the benign status of an erosion, a D & C should be performed also, to detect possible malignancy of the endocervix and corpus.

Before biopsy, the Schiller test can be used to locate abnormal tissue. When applied to the cervix, aqueous iodine solution (Lugol's iodine) stains normal glycogenated squamous epithelium brown. In contrast, columnar epithelium as well as areas where epithelium is absent, or abnormal, growing, or atrophic squamous epithelium take on a bright yellow stain.

Although it has not gained wide acceptance in the United States, colposcopy can be used to detect surface abnormalities in the cervix. It consists of binocular visualization of the cervix under a bright light with at least 10 or 20 times magnification. Colpomicroscopy, a more recent development, magnifies the cervical portion about 700 times.

How Should Erosion Be Treated?

The best argument for treating benign erosion of the cervix is that treatment reduces the chances of carcinoma developing later in life. A less compelling argument is that it eliminates annoying discharge or bleeding.

In my experience, douches, local enzyme preparations, and styptics and caustics such as silver nitrate are not often helpful. On the other hand, office or hospital *electrocauterization* does usually effectively eliminate erosion; traditionally, most postpartum erosions are treated by cauterization. But the *coning biopsy* is still more valuable because it is both diagnostic and therapeutic: the whole area is made available for histologic evaluation and the site heals in with squamous epithelium. *Cervical amputation* is excellent therapy when the cervix is also greatly hypertrophied. When complicated by corporeal lesions, complete hysterectomy is indicated.

Differentiation between cervical erosion and early carcinoma should be done by a Papanicolaou smear and, when feasible, a biopsy of some sort. Even benign erosions should be treated to eradicate areas of reddening. Electrocautery and surgery are more effective than local medication.

QUESTIONS AND ANSWERS

Q. *Can a benign cervical erosion be considered a "normal" cervical change?*

A. Yes, if the columnar epithelium is congenitally on the portio, it may be considered merely "misplaced." If benign, it will recede into the canal in time.

Q. *Does a vaginitis cause a cervical erosion?*

A. No, not if by "erosion" we mean an area of columnar epithelium. According to the theory of Robert Meyer, however, inflammation leads to a superficial ulceration of squamous epithelium and columnar epithelium grows over the defect. The fact that squamous (rather than columnar) epithelium grows back when the cervix is cauterized or cut away casts doubt on this theory.

LUMPS IN THE BREAST

The woman of today is very much aware of the possible significance of a breast lump, an attitude which is commendable. Many examine their breasts at regular intervals and promptly report any suspicious area to their doctor. All of this is praiseworthy if it does not result in cancerphobia or in unwarranted breast biopsy.

The consistency of breast tissue varies widely from one patient to another; moreover, in the individual patient, it varies with age, menstruation, pregnancy, and lactation. Fully one-quarter of adult women at some time have irregular areas in their breasts, which might be called lumps but which are actually false masses. In contrast, a true lump or mass is much less common and may signify serious disease. How can one distinguish between a false mass and a true mass?

The False Mass

A false mass is more apparent on palpation if examined between the thumb and fingers, in contrast to a true mass, which is best detected by palpation. Although it has been referred to as a disease (chronic mastitis, cystic disease, or dysplasia), it is only a variation from the normal and a common one since it affects 25% of adult women. Irregularities produced by hyperplasia and involution that occur with each menses are most apparent just before menstruation, the time that women seem most inclined to examine their breasts. Typical irregularities are shown in Figure 1. "A" represents the "normal" breast just before menstruation when granularity or fine nodularity may be palpated (particularly in the upper outer quadrants) due to the lobular distention.

Illustration "A" is also typical of the intermenstrual breast of the 25% of women who have persistently irregular tissue. In their premenstrual phase, these breasts may resemble "B." Notice the many irregular false masses. You can tell they are false masses because the three dimensions are unequal; particularly they lack depth. They tend to form nodular, rope-like, discoid, or plaque-like structures, and are often bilateral. Length and breadth are unequal in contrast to neoplasms

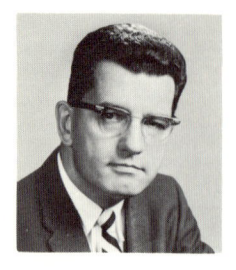

R. Cameron Harrison, M.D.
University of Alberta

Doctor Harrison is Professor of Surgery at the University of Alberta Faculty of Medicine. He is a Diplomate of the American Board of Surgery, Chairman of the Cancer Committee of the Canadian Medical Association, and a member of several other societies including the Royal College of Physicians and Surgeons (Canada), the American College of Surgeons, and the Canadian Association of Clinical Surgeons.

and cysts, which are about equal in all three dimensions. Women with false masses require only reassurance that their breasts are just "firmer than average." Reassurance is nullified if they are told they have cystic disease.

If the patient is premenopausal or menstruating, a suspicious lesion should be re-examined in two weeks; it is surprising how a worrisome area can lose its significance during that interval. If you are still in doubt, obtain a second opinion or proceed with biopsy.

Figure 1C illustrates one of the common causes of a true or dominant mass, the gross cyst. A gross cyst usually develops in an area of breast nodularity and there are often other areas of nodularity or granularity in the same or opposite breast. The smooth cyst wall presents as a dome in contrast to carcinoma, which has a more irregular surface. The cyst is more moveable for its size than carcinoma and is, of course, less hard. Fluctuation can rarely be elicited. Unless the axilla is heavily involved, examining it is not helpful in the differential diagnosis between benign and malignant disease.

The earliest sign of fixation, which is characteristic of carcinoma, is dimpling of the skin when it is molded over the lesion. It is most easily detected under oblique light. Just reduce the natural elasticity of the skin overlying the lesion by placing the thumb and forefinger on either side of the lump; then move your thumb and finger closer together. If the lesion is carcinoma,

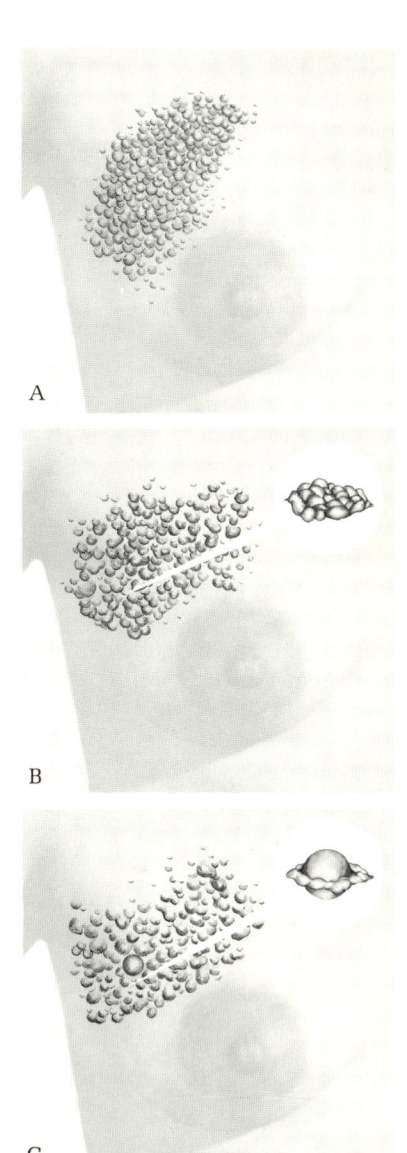

Figure 1—Artist's conception of the way various lumps within the breast feel upon palpation. A. Fine granularity in the upper outer quadrant. B. A false mass produced by coarse granularity. C. A cyst within the granular area.

you should see dimpling unless the lesion is extremely small or deep. Dimpling also occasionally occurs in very superficial benign lesions, plasma cell mastitis, and fat necrosis.

Finally, suspect a fibroadenoma in young women when the mass is well circumscribed. Extreme mobility is its most characteristic feature; when palpated, it tends to escape from under your fingers. These three lesions, cysts, carcinoma and fibroadenoma, constitute 95% of all true masses.

Treatment of the True Mass

All true masses must be investigated further. Unless you suspect that the lesion is a cyst, this means a biopsy and quick section under general anesthesia with facilities at hand for immediate mastectomy if carcinoma is found. To delay the mastectomy is unfair because it means putting the patient under anesthesia twice within a few days. Moreover, if a hematoma or infection should develop in the wound, mastectomy would be greatly delayed. However, if the lesion resembles a cyst, you can safely aspirate it in your office under local anesthesia.

To do so, the cyst must be 1.5 centimeters or larger, large enough to be located with a needle. All equipment must be within reach, because you must steady the mass between the left thumb and index finger while holding the syringe in the right hand. With a No. 20 needle, infiltrate the skin with a small amount of anesthetic; then attach a 10 cc. syringe and insert the needle into the mass. You will feel considerable resistance when the needle encounters the cyst; at this time hold the barrel of the syringe outward to produce a slight negative pressure. Advance the needle into the cyst, and aspirate the contents while applying pressure with the left thumb and index finger. If the volume exceeds 10 cc., leave the needle in place, empty the syringe, and complete the aspiration.

This simple treatment is all that is needed if (1) no residual mass remains after aspiration, (2) no blood is found in the aspirated fluid, and (3) the mass has not recurred when you examine the breasts three and six weeks later. Unless all three criteria are satisfied, open biopsy under general anesthesia with facilities for quick section is indicated. Surprisingly, most cysts do not recur, although new cysts often develop elsewhere in the breasts after either aspiration or excision.

Thus, the important first step in the management of a lump in the breast is to separate the true mass from the false. A true mass requires biopsy under general anesthesia and frozen section. The exception is the cyst, which can be aspirated in your own office under local anesthetic.

DYSMENORRHEA

As a rule, the human body expels waste painlessly. The one frequent exception to the rule is menstruation. Why should the expulsion of endometrial debris from a seemingly healthy uterus be painful for so many women?

The number and variety of explanations offered for dysmenorrhea are a testimony to our lack of understanding of the underlying cause. Although complete understanding may be years away, we already know some things about the uterine physiology of dysmenorrhea — things that help us to understand why pain occurs and, more important clinically, to suggest a practical treatment. But before discussing treatment, let me review some physiology.

First of all, recall that pain invariably arises when any hollow viscus expels a substance disproportionately large for its lumen. Specifically, primary dysmenorrhea arises when the uterus must expel a disproportionately large quantity of endometrial debris. This explains why patients with dysmenorrhea usually say their cramps are relieved just as soon as they pass the "clots," i.e., the endometrial fragments. It also explains why dysmenorrhea occurs only after ovulation, when the endometrium is thick, succulent, and hyperemic, and hence the quantity of material expelled is great. Conversely, a hollow viscus that readily accommodates its contents expels it painlessly. Thus, in the absence of organic disease, the relatively thin endometrium in the proliferative phase of the anovulatory cycle is nearly always expelled painlessly.

Furthermore, we know that myometria vary in their capacity to accommodate large amounts of debris. In women with dysmenorrhea, the myometria can stretch relatively little without pain. We can show this by using an intrauterine balloon to stretch the myometrium until the woman feels the characteristic pain of dysmenorrhea. Women who habitually menstruate painlessly tolerate distension as great as 7 cc. without pain. Women who habitually menstruate painfully tolerate as little as 2 cc. to 2.5 cc. without pain.

Finally, women with dysmenorrhea have a characteristically disordered pattern of myometrial contractions. Intrauterine balloon studies

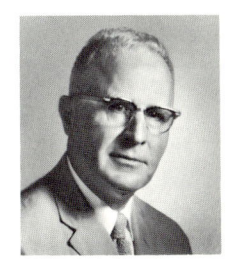

William Bickers, M.D.
American University of Beirut, Lebanon

Doctor Bickers is Professor and Chairman of Obstetrics and Gynecology at the American University of Beirut in Beirut, Lebanon. He is a member of the American Association for the Advancement of Science, the American Society for the Study of Sterility, and the South Atlantic Association of Obstetricians and Gynecologists. He has written two books, CLINICAL GYNECOLOGY and MENORRHALGIA: MENSTRUAL DISTRESS.

show that, in women who menstruate painlessly, the myometrium contracts in orderly, rhythmic waves that sweep debris toward the cervix. In women with dysmenorrhea, the contractions are disordered and hypertonic.

Apparently, then, pain occurs when the endometrial debris to be expelled is large and the capacity of the myometrium to stretch is limited and its contractions disordered. Pain may also occur when the endometrial debris is normal but must be excreted by a diseased uterus. For example, adenomyosis or intramural fibroids impair the ability of the myometrium to accommodate even normal amounts of debris.

What Is the Best Treatment for Dysmenorrhea?

Dysmenorrhea is a common complaint; perhaps half of all women suffer some discomfort during their menstrual periods. But in only 5% or 10% is the discomfort severe enough to require treatment; even these usually respond to simple analgesics. A few, however, suffer disabling symptoms and need intensive treatment.

This treatment may be directed at two targets: the endometrium and the myometrium. First, the amount of endometrial debris to be excreted can be reduced by any drug that suppresses ovulation, for this changes the normal secretory endometrium to a proliferative one. Since the amount of debris from an anovulatory proliferative endometrium is small, suppression of ovulation is followed by painless menstruation. Second, suppressing ovulation increases the vascularity and improves the contractions of the myometrium. If we establish orderly contractions capable of efficiently expelling the endometrial debris, and if the myometrium relaxes well between contractions, menstruation should be painless.

Both objectives are met by the use of steroids to induce a state of pseudopregnancy. This state is remarkably like a normal pregnancy except for the absence of placenta, fetus, and excretion of chorionic gonadotropin. The myometrium enlarges and undergoes deciduation, which reaches its peak during the third month of treatment. Breasts enlarge and lactation may follow steroid withdrawal. All these changes are caused by inducing a persistent progestational phase like that normally induced by the corpus luteum of pregnancy. Since normal pregnancy cures primary dysmenorrhea, is it not logical to use a pseudopregnancy to do the same thing?

Pseudopregnancy causes hypertrophy in the myometrium, the dry weight of the uterus being increased about 18% during seven months of steroid therapy. This myometrial growth associated with increased vascular and lymphatic supply favors a more orderly contraction pattern during the menstruation that follows progesterone therapy. The amplitude of the contractions increases and between contractions the myometrium relaxes completely. After steroid therapy, the myometrium better accommodates the mass within.

Moreover, the disordered gradient of intracavitary pressures from fundus to cervix that occurs under estrogen influence is altered by progesterone. Under progesterone influence, the ordered regular contractions favor an intracavitary gradient highest at the fundus and lowest at the cervix, thus encouraging the rapid and painless evacuation of menstrual debris.

What Is the Treatment Schedule?

Start treatment on the fifth day of the cycle using increasing doses of norethynodril or one of the other steroids now available. Give 10 mg. of norethynodril daily for the first month, 20 mg. daily during the second month, 30 mg. the third month, 40 mg. the fourth month, 50 mg. the fifth month.* If, at any time during the five months, breakthrough bleeding occurs, immediately increase the dose by 10 mg. and add subsequent monthly increases to that level. (An alternative schedule is the intramuscular injection of 100 mg. of injectable medroxyprogesterone every two weeks.) Be sure to continue the treatment for at least 6 to 7 months. Stopping during the second or third month may cause profuse uterine hemorrhage because this is the time of maximum proliferation and deciduation of a very vascular endometrium. Only after the third month will hyalinization, regression, and fibrosis begin; thereafter, stopping the drug is followed by normal menstruation.

For the most part, the side effects are negligible. As in pregnancy, headache, nausea, and vomiting may trouble some patients, and the incidence of thrombosis in the leg veins may be greater than in nonpregnant women. Some patients complain of breast fullness, congestion, weight gain, and all of the other symptoms associated with a positive water balance. In approximately 15% of the patients, these symptoms are unpleasant enough to discontinue treatment. There is no evidence that permanently harmful effects follow steroid treatment. Some pathologists have become concerned by one or two reports of stroma reactions in the endometrium, but they have been reported only in older women who probably should not have been treated with steroids anyway.

If the treatment is carried on for seven months, you can expect relief of dysmenorrhea in the great majority of patients. The amount of uterine bleeding is usually less after treatment; whereas menstruation formerly may have lasted five or six days, it may now last only three or four days. Normal cyclic menstruation usually begins three to four weeks after discontinuing treatment. Pregnancy promptly occurs when there is an opportunity for fertilization.

---

* These doses exceed those recommended by the manufacturer.

PREMENSTRUAL TENSION

Premenstrual tension affects about 50% of all menstruating women. It usually begins with a feeling of mild anxiety, depression, or irritability about 7 to 14 days before menstruation. As menstruation nears, these personality changes increase, crescendo-like, to reach a peak shortly before menstruation. At this time, the marked depression, crying spells for no apparent cause, anxiety, apprehension, insomnia, marked fatigue or frenzied restlessness, disturbance in sex desire, and inability to concentrate or to cope with routine daily problems, create a pathetic picture. Following the onset of the menstrual flow the symptoms usually disappear dramatically.

Often, there are physical symptoms, too: painful swelling of the breasts, headache, edema, nausea, abdominal bloating and cramps, craving for special foods, and weight gain. However, these symptoms are not often particularly uncomfortable or alarming; many patients seem to accept them philosophically as woman's lot. At any rate, emotional symptoms are much more likely to cause patients to seek medical advice.

Severe premenstrual tension affects the patient's family and friends. The patient often flares up at her husband over some trivial or imagined slight; she may almost "jump out of her skin" when the baby whimpers; she may interpret the children's usual behavior as sadistic rebellion, may find fault with, and even withdraw from intimate friends, and may fear that she is going insane. The bewilderment and distress of her family during these unnerving changes can be compared only to their intense relief when the patient becomes her usual sunny self again, not realizing the havoc she has created.

You can be a great help to the family in such cases by explaining what is going on. Curiously enough, until you do, probably neither the patient nor her family will be aware of the cause of the disturbances despite their monthly recurrence.

On the other hand, if you are misled by the paucity of objective findings, you may inadvertently minimize the importance of their symptoms by a casual remark such as, "It's just your nerves." No wonder many

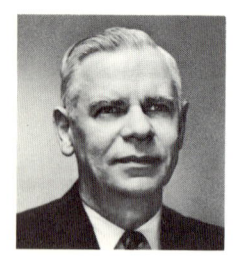

Joseph H. Morton, M.D.
New York City, New York

Doctor Morton specializes in endocrinology and psychosomatic medicine in New York City, and is Consultant in Endocrinology at South Nassau Communities Hospital in Oceanside, New York. For many years, he was a member of the research and teaching staffs of New York Medical College, Flower and Fifth Avenue Hospitals, and Endocrine Consultant at Metropolitan Hospital.

women with premenstrual tension would rather have a broken leg! At least the cast would draw some sympathy.

Social Effects

Premenstrual tension also takes a toll by curbing productivity, contributing to accidents, and in extreme cases, provoking antisocial behavior. These three social effects are illustrated by the following three cases.

The first woman, a factory worker with premenstrual tension, is clumsy and irritable on the job and sometimes unable to work at all; the result is a slowdown of her entire production line. A second woman, driving her automobile while jittery, tense, and exhausted by the functional hypoglycemia so commonly noted in premenstrual tension, fails to see a red light and crashes into a stopped car in front of her. The role of premenstrual tension in accidents is rarely suspected. Third, a teenage girl, who is well-behaved three weeks out of four, may repeatedly fight with friends and family during her premenstrual week. I know of one such girl who even ran away from home and eventually ended up in reform school.

Premenstrual tension undoubtedly contributes to antisocial behavior more often than we realize. Our studies in a large women's prison demonstrated that social attitude, behavior, and work output were adversely affected during the premenstrual period. Inmates were more irritable and pugnacious, broke more rules, demanded more analgesics and sedatives, could not maintain average work production, and required more disciplinary action. Several inmates repeatedly requested to be isolated during these days to avoid punishment for their compulsive acts and to avoid marring their records for the parole board. We found that 62% of unpremeditated crimes of violence (murder, manslaughter, and assault) were committed in the premenstrual week and 17% during early menstruation.

Individualized Treatment

As yet, no single drug or therapy completely alleviates or prevents premenstrual tension. Treatment should vary according to the patient's symptoms.

Superficial psychotherapy — The value of explanation and reassurance is demonstrated by the fact that 15% to 20% of patients respond to placebos. Only rarely, when serious depressive or suicidal tendencies are suspected, or when the patient does not respond to combined medical treatment and psychotherapy, is psychiatric consultation necessary.

Diet and drugs — Prescribe a high-protein, low-salt diet with frequent feedings to minimize functional hypoglycemia and fluid retention. Drugs should be prescribed for the particular individual's symptoms. Therefore, any of the following may be used: analgesics, diuretics, vitamins, tranquilizers, antispasmodics, and antidepressants. Hormones are of little value unless there is some underlying endocrine dysfunction, such as hyperthyroidism or hypometabolism. The unwise use of hormones may even disrupt the normal balance.

We have obtained dramatic results with the intravenous injection of 5 to 20 mg. of methamphetamine hydrochloride in severe premenstrual tension. Within a minute or two, a sudden easing of tension and depression occurs, with a subsequent increase in energy and a decrease in fatigue. Intravenous methamphetamine may also be useful as a prehypnotic antispasmodic to facilitate the induction of the hypnotic trance.

Treating associated disorders — Severe premenstrual tension is frequently aggravated by some other condition, such as hyperthyroidism, hypometabolism, obesity, chronic cystic mastitis, menstrual disturbances, neuroses, and psychoses.

QUESTIONS AND ANSWERS

Q. *What is the cause of the symptoms in premenstrual tension?*

A. Despite its high incidence and widespread serious effects, the exact cause of premenstrual tension is still obscure. Most investigators believe that an estrogen-progesterone imbalance with a relative excess of estrogen causes a retention of sodium with a subsequent increase in extracellular fluid. The uninhibited premenstrual estrogenic rise is also believed to increase sugar tolerance. This readily explains some of the psychic symptoms, including the heightened anxiety and fatigue. I have seen patients who show a flat or low sugar tolerance curve with a drop in the fourth or fifth hour during the premenstrual period and a normal sugar tolerance curve in the postmenstrual period.

Q. *Is hypnosis indicated in the management of premenstrual tension?*

A. The judicious use of hypnotherapy often produces a dramatic lessening of tension and depression. But, unless you are psychiatrically oriented and well trained in the use of hypnosis, you should avoid any deep uncovering techniques, which may create or enhance strong hostility and aggression in women with poor acceptance of the feminine role.

MENOPAUSAL COMPLAINTS
Practical Management

Grow old along with me!
The best is yet to be,
The last of life, for which
the first was made...
— ROBERT BROWNING

I have been engaged in the fields of medical education, research in the physiology of reproduction, and treatment of sexual problems for nearly 40 years, and during this time have dealt with (or tried to deal with) nearly every medical problem you can think of. Looking back, one problem stands out above all others for its prevalence (it affects half the population), for its variability (it affects some patients more severely than others), for its vagueness (some doctors call it a disease, others don't), and for its needless toll in apprehension, dread, and suffering: menopause. Even as a boy, I had heard about the "change of life." This was a supposedly dangerous and painful period of transition, and the very name itself conjured up the impression that every woman had to endure four or five years of suffering to become transformed and aged, withered, like a grape into a raisin.

Nowadays, of course, we know that menopause is not all that serious, that it is no more a disease than puberty is. But, it still remains a problem, and I think it does because it happens to occur at a time of life fraught with problems anyway — social, medical, and psychological problems. Even if the ovaries could go on functioning during these "difficult years," we would probably see just as many middle-aged women in our offices with just about the same complaints. Let us examine menopause in light of this concept, to see what the main problems are and, more important, what you can do about them.

Problem 1: The Dread of Growing Old

In contrast to puberty, which every child welcomes as a sign of growing older, menopause is universally unwelcome as a sign of growing *old*.

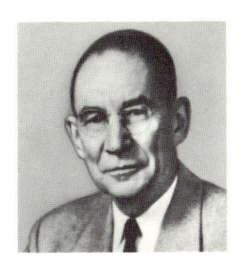

G. Lombard Kelly, M.D.
Augusta, Georgia

Doctor Kelly is President Emeritus and Professor Emeritus of Anatomy of the Medical College of Georgia, and formerly a Research Associate in Anatomy, Cornell Medical School. He is a Charter Member of the Society for the Scientific Study of Sex, and a member of the American Association of Anatomists. His publications include a well-known marriage manual distributed through physicians.

Few women, if any, look forward to it, because of all the signs of growing old, it is the surest. It is the one sign that cannot be disbelieved, cannot be explained away nor blamed on other things. Actually, of course, nature is probably wise to end a woman's reproductive years when it does — because it is a time when her body begins to age, when her strength diminishes, and when her health is really too precarious for her to begin raising a child.

To combat overconcern about this change — to combat waning vitality, real and imagined — and to reduce the likelihood of overweight, I prescribe exercises. I tell them to begin slowly and to gradually increase the number of exercises they do. To combat the common feeling of loss of femininity (which is more often unconscious than conscious) I advise my patients to pay special attention to hygiene and grooming . . . to take menopause as a good opportunity to spruce up a bit, try out new hair styles, modernize their wardrobe.

Remember, no matter how you do it, your main goal in managing menopausal patients is to combat their dread of aging.

Problem 2: Legitimate Symptoms of Estrogen Curtailment

One of the surprising things about menopause is that more women *don't* have troublesome symptoms as a result of the hormonal storm that occurs. After all, the curtailment of estrogen is a serious loss, considering that estrogen normally exerts so many different actions — maintaining blood supply, helping storage of protein for the development of muscle, and aiding in the use of calcium by the bones, to mention a few. In many surveys, and in my practice, the incidence of menopausal women who develop physical symptoms severe enough for them to seek treatment appears to be only about 10% to 15%. The chief symptom, vasomotor instability ("hot flushes"), is particularly disquieting to these women, and should always indicate the temporary use of hormone substitution treatment. Rarely will simple reassurance or sedation suffice. The attacks may be light or severe, and they can lead to discomfort and embarrassment. When they occur during sleep, vessel dilation may cause marked perspiration.

For this symptom, estrogen should be given, in small oral doses on a definite cyclic schedule so that if withdrawal bleeding occurs, it can be reasonably attributed to the treatment and not to an unrecognized uterine malignancy. I usually give estrogen for 30 days, stop for seven days, then resume this cycle. Most patients can be weaned away from the hormone in a few months. I do not agree with those who advocate prolonged use of replacement therapy, or with those who believe replacement therapy should be given to every menopausal woman. To my mind, there is no point in delaying the inevitable physical adjustment that menopause requires; to maintain a woman on estrogen indefinitely makes no more sense than to start a 7-year-old girl on estrogen. Only when the symptoms make it a necessity should it be given.

The other typical symptoms of menopause — nervousness, irritability, anxiety, fatigue, insomnia, and general aches and pains — should not always be attributed immediately to hormonal curtailment, and can often be treated individually by means other than hormonal replacement. One point to remember is that fatigue, when it occurs in menopausal patients, may be a symptom of some serious disease such as diabetes or heart disease, and should lead you to do a thorough physical and laboratory examination.

There are many other symptoms said to be due to the menopause, but I do not consider them significant: abnormal rapidity of the heart, difficulty in breathing, decreased memory and concentration, blind spots in the visual field, digestive disturbances, nausea, mild indigestion, tingling of the skin, numbness of the extremities, frequency of urination, and coldness of the extremities. The only treatment they require is reassurance of the patient that they are transient and harmless.

Problem 3: The Happenstance Co-existence of Other Disorders

As we all know, the incidence of many diseases climbs during middle age, and many of these reach a peak about the time of menopause. According to U.S. Public Health reports, for example, hypertension and arteriosclerosis are nearly 10 times more prevalent at age 45 than at age 20; gastric and duodenal ulcer are 5 times more prevalent.

Many of the so-called problems of menopause probably stem from the co-existence of these disorders and the toll they take in general health. Look for tuberculosis (a common cause of fatigue), and for diabetes (a source of some bizarre symptoms). Remember to check for glaucoma, and also for dental problems, which begin to multiply during this time. And finally, check for cancer and instruct your patients how to examine their breasts for cancer, if they do not know how.

If we do these things, if we consider menopause as a good opportunity to practice preventive medicine, we may greatly benefit our patients.

Problem 4: The Threat to Stability

Most women can take menopause in stride, but some cannot (or do not) because of the intense emotional problems it stirs up. Usually, in such cases, the woman was prone to them anyway, and the stress of menopause merely poured gasoline on a smouldering fire. Consider, for example, the following case:

Mrs. E. C., a 46-year-old woman, came to my attention through her sister, who had called me about her. Mrs. C. had been highly neurotic all of her life and had accepted the sexual obligation of marriage with reluctance and with complete absence of pleasure or gratification; menstruation had often been painful for her, and she disliked it intensely. Only one child blessed the union, now at 26 a capable, rising attorney with a promising future. Only the father's deep love and affection for this son had kept the marriage together. Now with the son's imminent marriage and jealousy of the prospective daughter-in-law, Mrs. C. feared an early dissolution of her marital status and social position.

Added to the foregoing, the deeply religious convictions of Mrs. C. intensified her problems. The common symptoms of the menopause in this woman were severe. Fortunately, the husband, the son and his fiancee were all most sympathetic and they succeeded in persuading the patient to accept in a spirit of full cooperation the indicated medical advice and treatment. A marked improvement was soon evident and continued to what might be termed a satisfactory recovery. Much credit must be given to capable assistance from a highly qualified psychiatrist and to an understanding and sympathetic minister in whom the devout sufferer had the utmost confidence.

This case touches on some of the more important ramifications of menopause. First of all, the woman had always held a puritanical attitude towards sex and had never completely accepted the feminine role. Her life-long abhorrence of menstruation had not made menopause easier, and her other problems made it more stormy. Women such as this are sometimes difficult to help, and our best lesson from them is what we can do to prevent similar situations in the future. Girls should be better prepared for romance, marriage, and childbearing, so that they can accept each step as it comes. They should know more about what makes a woman a woman and a man a man, so that they can build a better and more stable marriage. They should be taught to cultivate hobbies and interests outside the home, to put their eggs in several baskets. Such activities not only give a woman a sense of self-esteem but can also enable her to accept the menopause without concern.

When faced with such a case, I always remember one axiom: *idleness is the worst enemy of emotional stability during the menopausal transition.* Worries multiply when someone sits with folded hands and lets her mind wander. Think of the possible things that you can suggest for a woman to do to keep active.

Problem 5: Failure to Recognize What's Good About Menopause

Finally, one approach to managing menopausal patients (and one that I think works best) is to communicate to your patients the idea that there are many good things about it. I realize that this is easier said than done,

and that it requires ingenuity. My reasoning, though, is based on the belief that if we physicians consider menopause as a disease, we are bound to magnify our patients' symptoms and make patients think it is, too. Mild transient symptoms that ought to be ignored, if examined in the light of serious concern, tend to become serious. Instead, I believe we should try to adopt a positive attitude toward menopause.
* It is a good time to take stock of one's life, to plan ahead for better things — grandchildren (which they can enjoy without work), new activities, long-postponed associations.
* It is a time when, if the children have gone, a woman can participate with her husband in activities like golfing and traveling, or even possibly in business ventures.
* It is a good time to try new things: painting, sculpting, writing, or anything she has always wanted to try — but never had time for.
* For some women, menopause is a good time to go back to work.
* For most women, it means a relief to dispense with pads or tampons. It will certainly mean relief for those who have suffered from endometriosis with its discomforts, painful intercourse, and other complications.

* * *

To help menopausal patients, then, requires ingenuity and patience. Perhaps I can sum up my philosophy about menopause — and the one I try to impart to my patients — by the following quotation from the English educator, Thomas Arnold (1794-1842):

Probably the happiest period of life is in middle age, when the eager passions of youth are cooled, and the infirmities of age not yet begun . . . as we see that the shadows, which are at morning and evening so large almost entirely disappear by midday.

MENOPAUSAL COMPLAINTS
Hormonal Management

The human ovary is an example of a vital organ that dies well in advance of its owner. Curiously, *Homo sapiens* is the only species that undergoes this phenomenon; in lower animals, ovarian life expectancy and general life expectancy coincide. As you will see from the arguments that follow, I believe that *Homo sapiens* is no better equipped than any other species to live one-third of a lifetime without the important ovarian hormones.

Pro and Con

I would be perfectly willing to adopt, for the sake of discussion, the point of view that the menopause is a pathologic rather than a physiologic phenomenon. What could possibly sustain such a point of view? For one thing, most of the contemporary studies of the metabolic effects of the steroids would indicate that it is harmful, rather than good, to lose such a major source of hormone complement. The rise in blood lipid levels and the rising incidence of coronary artery disease that follow the decline in estrogen levels certainly cannot be described as "good." The effects of negative protein balance, first the withdrawal of protein from the matrix of the bone and then calcium depletion of the long bones, is never beneficial: the 80-year-old lady who suffers a fractured hip can blame it, to some extent, on the fact that her ovaries ceased functioning 30 years before. The difficulty in salt retention (which, incidentally, makes sodium chloride such a helpful medication in geriatrics) is another index of the impact of this steroid withdrawal. The beneficial influence of sex steroid replacement on senile mental aberrations demonstrated by B. M. Caldwell suggests another area in which the postmenopausal population suffers from deprivation of these hormones.

These changes can hardly be described as beneficial, or even as "proper," and indeed it would be somewhat strange if one could lose such an important member of the interrelated family of endocrine glands as the ovary without some less-than-desirable side effects. The list of

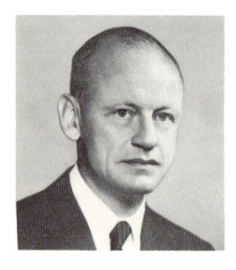

Allan C. Barnes, M.D.
Johns Hopkins University

Doctor Barnes is Professor and Chairman of the Department of Gynecology and Obstetrics of Johns Hopkins University School of Medicine. He is also an editor of the AMERICAN JOURNAL OF OBSTETRICS AND GYNECOLOGY. He is a Fellow of the American College of Surgeons and of the American College of Obstetricians and Gynecologists, and a member of the American Association of Obstetricians and Gynecologists.

such effects above is only partial, but remains sufficient for the moment to convince me that the menopause is a pathologic entity.

Now what is the argument in favor of assigning the menopause to the category of the *physiologic* rather than pathologic? There is, to the best of my knowledge, only one such argument: namely, that it happens to every woman. Neglecting a phenomenon medically simply because it is universal, of course, is unsound reasoning. Death is also universal, yet we struggle against it. My ophthalmologist, when I consulted him about the fact that telephone directories were obviously being printed in smaller and smaller type, did not reply: "Middle-age presbyopia is universal; it happens to everyone; therefore, I shall not treat it by giving you glasses." Fortunately he has intelligence and wrote me the proper prescription.

The general practitioner or gynecologist with equal intelligence (and compassion) can likewise treat the menopause. As an excuse for nontreatment, universality of occurrence is not a satisfactory argument whether dealing with optic failure or with ovarian failure. Therefore, in my practice, the menopause is a disease process, requiring active intervention. The idea is not new, of course, and has been practiced and advocated by many more eloquent than I.

Treatment of the Menopause

The first of the hazards such practice encounters is that the replacement of ovarian steroids with estrogens alone can often lead to uterine bleeding complications. (Carcinogenesis as a threat is largely armchair reasoning, and E. K. Shelton's thorough study would seem to have ruled this out.) This threat of uterine bleeding is removed if the estrogen is given with an androgen.

The work of A. M. Shearman and others would indicate that the best ratio of methyltestosterone to diethylstilbestrol is 20:1. Certainly his figures in support of this ratio are impressive, and the therapeutic impact on osteoporosis, mental depression, urinary tract symptoms, etc., is much greater from the androgen component than from the estrogenic component. However, since we are using it for prevention rather than therapy, we shall settle for a 10:1 ratio, which will still maintain a quiescent, nonbleeding endometrium. The actual dose would be 5 mg. of methyltestosterone and 0.5 mg. of stilbestrol daily, omitting the first four to six days of each calendar month. The patient should remain on this program until she is 86, an age I cite only to impress upon her the long-continued need for the steroid supplement. Like the patient who has a deficiency state and needs insulin now, she is also going to need it just as much ten or fifteen years from now.

Actually the true threat of such therapy is that the physician will relax and think that these medicines have "fixed everything." Medicine postpones and delays some of the manifestations of the postmenopausal state, but it does not relieve the physician from his responsibility to be a sympathetic counsellor and firm advisor. Nutritional counselling and an adjustment of the height-weight ratio is important. Regular check-up examinations are imperative; there is nothing in this regimen to produce immunity to cervical or ovarian malignancy. Preventive psychotherapy should have started at least a decade before; now psychotherapy should be intensified.

The present plea, in other words, is not that we substitute steroid replacement for all other forms of management of the menopausal patient, but that we include the proper steroid replacement along with the other forms. As our general health measures improve and life expectancy increases, we face the probability that the number of decades that a woman will outlive her ovaries will increase. Unless this serious deficiency is replaced, these will be decades of unnecessarily rapid degeneration. I say, the postmenopausal state is a disease requiring our active treatment.

QUESTIONS AND ANSWERS

Q. *When during menopause do you begin steroid treatment?*

A. I prefer to wait until the patient has been amenorrheal for at least six months. However, if she complains of uncomfortable menopausal symptoms such as hot flashes, I sometimes begin treatment as early as two months after her last period.

Q. *A woman of 65 registers in your practice for the first time. She says she passed through the menopause without difficulty at the age of 55. She is now untroubled by menopausal symptoms. Would you start her on a program of steroid replacement?*

A. If the patient is presumably going to remain in my practice for her gynecologic check-ups and guidance, I would start her on the above program. I would explain its nature and purpose and try to assure myself that she would be reasonably faithful about such a prolonged program of medication. If she understood my motivation and seemed willing to cooperate, I would certainly initiate this program. The fact that she is asymptomatic, of course, would not deter me. I am not at the moment as interested in symptoms as I am in "chemical balance."

INTRACTABLE INFECTIOUS VAGINITIS

Infectious vaginitis may severely tax the physician's ingenuity and patience. Of course, it often responds to simple, more or less nonspecific measures. But what about the frustrating, intractable case — the kind that each of us encounters all too often? Why does it seem to resist all treatment?

Treatment of vaginal infections fails for one or more of the following reasons: (1) incorrect initial diagnosis, (2) unrecognized change in diagnosis during treatment, (3) incorrect treatment, (4) inadequate intensity or duration of treatment, (5) reinfection, or (6) overtreatment.

Need for Accurate Diagnosis

I have chosen to discuss conditions that are not likely to respond to "shot gun" therapy. By definition, then, successful management depends upon discovering the specific cause or causes; it depends upon careful history-taking, pelvic examination, and laboratory tests. Moreover, these three steps should be repeated at every office visit to evaluate the effect of treatment or possible change of etiology.

Important in history-taking is the time of onset of the symptoms, the course of the disease, and the treatment so far. Note the nature (amount, color, and odor) of the discharge. Also ask the patient if she has experienced pruritus, local edema, dyspareunia, soreness, or external burning when urinating. Discharge is the predominant symptom of trichomoniasis; pruritus is more often the predominant symptom of candidiasis.

Pelvic examination should be complete and thorough, whether the patient is pregnant or not. The purpose is to assess the extent and the type of vaginitis, but you should also be alert for more serious concomitant disease. *Trichomonas vaginalis* vaginitis causes vaginal inflammation with a greenish profuse, purulent, malodorous, bubbly discharge. *Candida* (monilial) vulvovaginitis causes a scanty, highly irritating discharge with white flecks. The vaginal epithelium is reddened with white ("cream cheese" or "cottage cheese") patches; the vulva may be inflamed with local edema. In cases of atrophic vaginitis, the

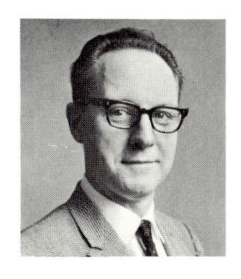

Warren R. Lang, M.D.
Jefferson Medical College

Doctor Lang is a Professor of Obstetrics and Gynecology at Jefferson Medical College of Philadelphia. He is also Associate Director of Obstetrics, and Chief of the Vaginitis Clinic, at Jefferson Medical College Hospital. He has served as chairman of several conferences of the New York Academy of Sciences, and as editor of the transactions of the Inter-Society Cytology Council. He is Secretary-Treasurer of the American Society of Cytology.

epithelium is thin, inflamed, and occasionally ulcerated. Bacterial vaginitis, which is rare in my experience, shows merely inflammation clinically.

Of all the laboratory tests useful in the diagnosis of vaginitis, the most informative and the easiest to perform is the wet smear. Simply wipe the posterior fornix with a cotton-tipped applicator, and insert the cotton with its specimen of vaginal secretions into a test tube containing a milliliter of physiologic saline solution. Place a drop under the microscope, and look for the following: epithelial cells (parabasal or squamous), motile trichomonads, hyphae indicative of *Candida*, leukocytes, erythrocytes, bacteria, spermatozoa, and debris. The average case of vaginal infection is easily diagnosed by this technique.

The Gram-stained smear permits a rough determination of vaginal microorganisms. For exact diagnosis and for an accurate evaluation of treatment, culture secretions for trichomonads, fungi, and bacteria. Papanicolaou smears are helpful in determining estrogen effect in the noninflamed vagina and in screening for malignancy. All suspicious lesions should be biopsied. Nonpregnant women with candidiasis should always be checked for diabetes mellitus.

General Principles of Therapy

Even though specific therapies are always desirable and necessary, there are certain general principles of management applicable to all varieties of vaginitis. Systemic measures play a minor role, except when systemic disease is present, too; for instance, candidiasis is frequently associated with diabetes mellitus, pregnancy, or the use of broad-spectrum antibiotics. Two other nonspecific measures that are occasionally helpful for trichomoniasis are treating the abnormal cervix, and excising the Skene's tubules. Only rarely has either proved useful in my experience. Also of little value, in my opinion, are efforts to thicken the epithelium (estrogen), to favor normal flora (introduction of *Lactobacilli*), to modify pH toward the acid side (various buffers), and to increase vaginal sugars (introduction of simple carbohydrates). Urologic investigation and treatment of the husband are recommended in intractable cases of trichomoniasis, however.

Management of Four Major Types of Vaginitis

Trichomonas vaginalis vaginitis is a chronic, recurrent, and resistant infection. Systemic treatment is certainly preferable to local treatment, since systemic treatment attacks the causative organism wherever it may be hiding. Metronidazole, a new oral medication, seems to be effective when administered to both wife and husband in dosages of

250 mg. three times daily for ten days. However, vaginal metronidazole given simultaneously does not seem to be necessary. Vaccines, so far, have failed.

Local medications should be administered over long periods but used with caution. I have had best results with diiodohydroxyquin 100 mg., an organic arsenical (Carbarsone®), and silver picrate. It should be remembered that arsenicals, although effective, may cause a dermatitis. Douching should be prescribed before insertion of this or any tablet. I prescribe a douche of lactic acid USP, 1 teaspoonful to two quarts of warm water.

Candida (monilial) vulvovaginitis is usually caused by *Candida albicans*. Local therapy is effective especially in nonpregnant women. I prefer nystatin tablets, chlordantoin cream, propionate compound jelly or a gentian violet compound. Sodium bicarbonate douches, 2 tablespoonfuls to two quarts of water, afford rapid relief at the onset of therapy. Vulvar itching, often associated with candidal vaginitis, is relieved by careful cleansing and applying nystatin powder or cool witch hazel compresses.

Bacterial vaginitis caused by mixed flora can be satisfactorily treated with lactic acid douches, triple sulfa vaginal tablets or cream, or nitrofurazone suppositories or cream. Cleansing douches suffice in mild cases. When specific bacterial infections such as *Staphylococcus aureus* are present, specific countermeasures determined by sensitivity testing are indicated.

Atrophic vaginitis can sometimes be relieved with mild douches or an acid-buffered jelly (Aci-Jel®); however, the atrophic vagina is frequently infected. Trichomoniasis and candidiasis infections are managed as described above. Estrogen creams are not usually required.

None of the foregoing comments is meant to suggest that treatment of infectious vaginitis can always succeed. However, careful, repeated diagnosis followed by persistent, specific treatment will conquer most seemingly intractable infections.

chapter 10

DIFFICULT-TO-MANAGE COMPLAINTS

HYPERTENSION THAT DEMANDS TREATMENT

Technically, a blood pressure above 160/90 mm. Hg is considered abnormal. Yet the question is often asked, "Which patients should be actively treated?" According to my experience, there are three groups that must be treated because of poor prognosis if left untreated: (1) men with diastolic hypertension, (2) patients with benign hypertension with familial history of malignant hypertension, and (3) all patients with malignant hypertension. I think the best way to describe these patients and their appropriate therapy is to relate three case histories, each one representing one of these three groups. Before doing that, however, I would like to put down some obvious but sometimes overlooked facts.

First, the essential parts of an examination to determine the severity of hypertension: familial and personal medical history, fundoscopic examination, chest X-ray, urinalysis, and blood urea nitrogen. For a reliable base line, repeated blood pressures should be recorded by the same person, at the same time of day, using the same equipment, on the same arm; and the examination should be done in an atmosphere of serenity and routine to avoid any emotional effect on blood pressure stemming from the procedure itself.

1. Men with Diastolic Hypertension

A 54-year-old laborer was admitted to the hospital complaining of severe occipital headache. For several years, he had noticed increasing dyspnea, and during the last six months had noticed daily swelling of the ankles. He did not have precordial pain. At examination, his blood pressure was 175/110 sitting and 186/114 recumbent. His heart was enlarged to the left as far as the anterior axillary line. He showed a 2 plus ankle edema and weighed 186 lbs. Lab tests showed a trace of albuminuria, specific gravity 1.018 (24-hour urine), normal CBC, and BUN 15 mg. per 100 ml. The EKG showed left ventricular hypertrophy confirmed by X-ray.

We began treatment with hydrochlorothiazide (50 mg. daily) and hydralazine (50 mg. t.i.d.). After four days, the blood pressure readings were down 20 points systolic and 14 diastolic. The patient now weighed

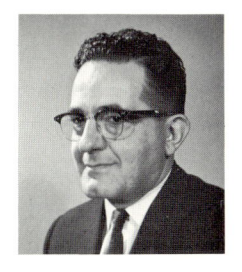

Benjamin Calesnick, M.D.
Hahnemann Medical College

Doctor Calesnick is Associate Professor of Pharmacology and Director of the Laboratory of Human Pharmacology at Hahnemann Medical College and also Chief of the Hypertension Clinic at St. Joseph's Hospital in Philadelphia. His professional affiliations include the American Society for Pharmacology and Experimental Therapeutics, and the Society of Nuclear Medicine.

182 lbs. He no longer complained of headache, but did complain of feeling more tired. So we reduced the hydrochlorothiazide to 25 mg. per day and supplemented his diet with 8 oz. of apricot juice daily. Within 48 hours, his fatigue subsided, but his blood pressure was unchanged. To reduce it further, we increased the hydralazine to 50 mg. q.i.d. One week later, his blood pressure was satisfactory at 146/92 sitting and 154/96 recumbent, and he was discharged on this regimen. Two weeks later, he was still comfortable. He weighed 180 lbs. and retained his previous reduction in blood pressure. He had only slight, pitting edema of the ankles, and the dyspnea, even at work, was markedly improved. He was considered stabilized at this point and was discharged for one month on the same regimen without limitation of salt intake. At the next examination he was, and still remains, well controlled and without gross complaints.

Comment — This case shows classic symptoms and physical and laboratory findings. It shows, too, that this kind of hypertension is readily controlled with a diuretic-antihypertensive combination. The occurrence of fatigue as a side effect and the varying response to different dosage levels of the drugs point up the need to adjust dosage carefully and individually in each patient.

2. Benign Hypertension with a Family History of Hypertension

A 37-year-old salesman was admitted to the hospital for cardiovascular evaluation. He had recently been denied life insurance because of familial hypertension: his father died of a stroke at 35 and his brother of coronary occlusion at 46. Sitting blood pressures recorded by the insurance medical examiner ranged between 168 to 185 systolic and 110 to 118 diastolic. His medical history was negative, except for the usual childhood diseases.

For the first four days, he was under continuous observation without antihypertensive medication. During this time, the recumbent blood pressure readings ranged between 118 to 132 (systolic) and 76 to 84 (diastolic). Pulse rate ran between 82 and 94. He weighed 156 lbs., and all laboratory tests including EKG, chest X-ray, and the histamine provocative test for pheochromocytoma were in the normal range.

We decided to discharge him on reserpine (0.25 mg. t.i.d.) and told him to return for an examination after one week. He returned complaining of severe nasal stuffiness and slight nausea. Blood pressure had risen 20 points above the maximum previously recorded. We then reduced the dosage to one tablet a day (0.25 mg.). The side effects still proved troublesome, however, so we discontinued it — replacing it with 30 mg. phenobarbital b.i.d. Two weeks later, he had no complaints, and the blood pressure readings were in the normal range (126/82 sitting and 132/84 recumbent). However, another month later, blood pressure was again in the hypertensive range. On questioning, he admitted that he had neglected to take his medication for the past three weeks because he thought he was "cured." His poor prognosis was again emphasized, especially in view of the family history, and he left, promising to continue on the medication. To date, he remains well controlled with mild sedation, but still needs continuous reminders about the need for treatment.

Comment — Such hypertension, in its early stages, is elusive and apparently benign. It produces no physical discomfort and may not even register on the sphygmomanometer, except sporadically. So, while it is quickly responsive to treatment with the mildest of sedatives, it presents a serious problem in that patients remain unconvinced of its importance and frequently progress to severe hypertension simply because of neglect. Perhaps the most important part of managing such patients is relentless follow-up.

3. Malignant Hypertension

A 59-year-old chauffeur was admitted to the hospital complaining of dyspnea, nocturia, fatigue, increasing blurring of vision, and headache which was present in the morning and grew progressively worse during the day. Blood pressures on admission were 240/124 recumbent and 232/128 standing; pulse was 120. He showed edema of both optic discs and retinal hemorrhage with sclerosis of the retinal arteries. The heart was enlarged to the left with EKG evidence of left axis deviation. Blood urea nitrogen was 27 mg. per 100 ml., urine showed a trace of albumin, and the phenolphthalein excretion in two hours was normal.

We began treatment with a ganglionic blocker, mecamylamine, 10 mg. b.i.d. After four days, blood pressure was slightly reduced but still over 200/100. His headaches were still present, so the dosage was increased to 12.5 mg. b.i.d. This produced further reduction to 205/102 recumbent and 160/84 standing (repeat BUN was 30 mg. per 100 ml.). However, he complained of marked constipation and some blurring of vision, and said he felt faint and lightheaded when standing. We decided at this point to give up ganglionic blockade and to attempt control of hypertension by chemical sympathectomy with guanethidine. At two-day intervals, we reduced the dosage of mecamylamine by 5 mg. per day and gradually increased the dosage of guanethidine by 5 mg. After 10 days, the patient was taking 25 mg. doses of guanethidine alone, twice a day. He was fairly comfortable on this regimen except for a mild diarrhea. After three days of stable blood pressure, we increased dosage to two 25 mg. tablets as a single dose after breakfast. After another week, the blood pressure began to rise again, so two more 25 mg. tablets were added to the daily dose. At this dosage the blood pressure appeared to be stabilized at 186/98 recumbent and 158/82 standing. The diarrhea was controlled with the addition of 5 mg. of homatropine. He was discharged from the hospital and followed in the clinic at biweekly intervals. His blood pressure remains reasonably stable, but dyspnea and headache still occur occasionally.

Comment — Hypertension of this severity responds only partially to any treatment and continues to progress in spite of repeated adjustments of doses and drugs. The best you can do is to get the blood pressure down as low as you can, and as soon as you can, with the least hazard and discomfort. Remember, however, that elevated blood pressure is just one symptom of hypertensive disease, and be wary of the natural temptation to concentrate just on rapid reduction of blood pressure. If it is reduced too abruptly, the effects of diminished renal, cerebral, and coronary blood flow may be even more harmful than the initial blood pressure. This is especially important in severe cases like patient No. 3. Such patients frequently develop renal failure as a result of diminished renal blood flow, and must be watched carefully for a rise in BUN. An important factor in avoiding precipitous changes in blood pressure is to make sure that all dosage changes and all withdrawals or substitutions of drugs are made gradually. Also, because treatment of these patients always involves very potent drugs, it is helpful to remember that there may be an advantage in combining several drugs with different sites of action; they may be synergistic and make possible smaller, and less toxic, doses of each drug.

Incidentally, an important precaution when prescribing a drug like guanethidine is to warn against the concomitant use of sympathomimetic drugs such as are commonly found in nose drops and asthma medication. Experimentally, the latter drugs' pressor effects are enhanced by guanethidine and related compounds; their concomitant use could cause the serious complications of an abrupt rise in blood pressure. One final point — about hypertensive crises, such as encephalopathy or acute cardiac insufficiency — I find that dramatic results can often be obtained with parenteral (I.V. or I.M.) reserpine (2.5 to 5.0 mg.) or hydralazine (20 to 40 mg.) every four to six hours.

In summary, then, the rule is: begin therapy with the mildest and safest drug which will produce the necessary lowering of blood pressure. Generally, I find it best to start treatment of the uncomplicated hypertensive with mild sedatives and tranquilizers such as reserpine and phenobarbital. In more severe cases, I add more potent (and more toxic) drugs in the following order: oral diuretics (thiazides); an arteriolar relaxant (hydralazine); chemical sympathectomy (guanethidine); and finally ganglionic blockers (chlorisondamine, pentolinium, mecamylamine) in carefully selected cases.

LOW-BACK PAIN

Most patients who want you to relieve low-back pain actually suffer from what I call the "low-back complex" — a lumbar spine derangement. This may produce local back pain with or without radiation. There are qualitative differences in the mechanism of the derangement and quantitative gradations within these categories. The overall plan of treatment is a progression from conservative measures to more specific local management.

This plan does not incorporate philosophy of trial and error but an awareness that the treatment should not be more rigorous than the effects of the condition. And, as the term low-back complex embraces more than one set of circumstances, there cannot be only one form of treatment for the condition. When pain is localized to the back, measures that reduce ligamentous inflammation and ease muscle spasm often provide relief; when pain radiation is a prominent feature, then its pattern can offer an understanding of its development and provide a key to more successful treatment.

Joint Parts at Fault

The low-back complex is a joint derangement brought about by a malfunction of the spinal muscle-ligament system; in short, sets of muscles that are supposed to work together smoothly somehow fail.

A derangement of the lumbar spine is a joint derangement. There are three parts to a true joint: First, the bearing surfaces and their enclosure — the synovia and capsule. Second, the fulcrum-establishment or stabilizing mechanism of the joint that maintains proper relationship of the bearing surfaces to each other. Third, the motor power that moves the joint or maintains the gross position of the two arms of the joint.

To appreciate the importance of a stable fulcrum, one has only to shut a heavy two-hinged door when one of the hinge pins is missing or a hinge plate is loose. Even though the bearing surfaces are intact and the motor power is adequate, the door will not close smoothly. To make up for the unstable fulcrum requires a substantial, awkwardly directed

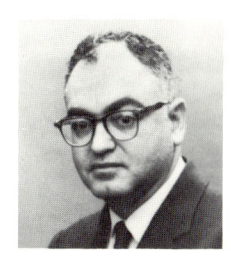

Harvey P. Kopell, M.D.
New York University

Doctor Kopell is Associate Professor of Orthopedic Surgery at New York University School of Medicine, and is active in the Neuro-Muscular Study Group at the New York University Bellevue Medical Center. He is associate visiting orthopedic surgeon, Bellevue Hospital, and assistant attending orthopedic surgeon, University Hospital. Doctor Kopell is a member of the American Academy of Orthopedic Surgeons.

motor power or force. Such a force may jam the door; jamming, in the case of joint motion, is akin to the effects produced by muscle spasm.

Joint Action of Spinal Muscles

Basically, two sets of muscles and associated ligaments control spinal movements. One, which binds only adjacent vertebrae together, acts to stabilize the fulcrum. The other — a larger group of muscles — crosses and joins several vertebrae to make up an articulated spinal segment and provide motor power to move it, or to maintain the position of the spinal column with relation to the pelvis and upper trunk.

The trouble comes when the set of motor muscles (muscles that cause gross movement) acts before the stabilizing group of muscles can provide a stable fulcrum. Jamming results. To make matters worse, the motor muscle unit then tries to take over to stabilize the fulcrum, but does not provide a proper force vector to maintain the bearing surfaces together. Abnormal joint motion results, which in turn may affect an intervertebral disc.

The disc, which acts like a shock absorber, serves to smooth out or limit the rate of joint movement. Fibers in its ring are in two groups which spiral in opposite directions and so cross each other along a vertical axis, somewhat like an Oriental finger trap. As in the finger trap, the fibers remain intact to a tensile, compressive, or torsional force, but tend to be deformed and weakened by shearing forces, which may result from faulty stabilization with inadequate muscular attempts at compensation.

Derangement of the overstressed or injured myoligamentous unit produces a local sterile inflammatory reaction which can cause pain. Abnormal motion which shears the joint adds to the distress.

Muscles that try to make up for the unstable fulcrum are another source of local pain. They work hard, but their direction of force is not exactly right to bring about stabilization, so spasm results. Spasm causes pain by exerting an abnormally strong pull against muscle attachments, or by producing a relative ischemia, because the spinal muscles do not have the intrinsic vascular status to maintain good circulation for continued contraction. The muscles that go into spasm cannot properly set or stabilize the joint; the direction of their force causes abnormal joint motion, which causes more pain and cyclically causes more spasm.

Localized Pain

Use of an anti-inflammatory agent, such as hydrocortisone, systemically or locally by infiltration, can allay inflammation in the deranged fulcrum-establishment mechanism.

Some mechanical disruption may persist because of compensatory muscle spasm, which in itself is painful and maintains the derangement. Spasm often perpetuates itself because the functional ischemia it produces increases both muscular irritability and stretch reflex. Spasm pain can be decreased by procaine infiltration or measures to stimulate circulation (heat, counterirritants, ethyl chloride spray). It can be attacked directly by muscle relaxants or by manipulative procedures that overload and temporarily inactivate the stretch reflex mechanism. Reducing the spasm, if it has aggravated the derangement, will ease the extra stress on the myoligamentous stabilization system, allowing it to recompensate to its prederangement state.

Radiating Pain

There are three basic causes of radiating pain associated with the low-back complex.

Pain associated with *irritated paraspinal structures* occurs at the attachment points of the spinal muscles and ligaments. Because of facilitation of pathway, the pain can be referred to a peripheral portion of the spinal segment. Therefore, a local spinal irritation can even cause sciatica. Pain of this sort should present no sensory deficit, motor atrophy, or reflex changes and can be relieved by infiltration of the paraspinal structures with a local anesthetic or an anti-inflammatory agent. The procedure here is both diagnostic and therapeutic. More than one injection may be needed and adjunctive treatment such as heat, muscle relaxants, and salicylates are useful. If such measures fail, then stabilization must be provided externally through a brace or internally by fusion.

In persons with a *herniated intervertebral disc,* pain and disability are usually referred to the terminal distribution of the affected nerve root. The resultant pain is soon accompanied by a radicular sensory deficit, motor weakness, and atrophy. When radiculopathy is not progressive, the patient often can be made comfortable by the usual adjunctive therapy, but when it is progressive, then laminectomy is necessary.

If local stabilization proves inadequate for the functional demands placed on the back after laminectomy, then fusion may be necessary.

Pain may be produced by *peripheral entrapment neuropathies* that develop in nerves that have an intimate relationship with muscles stabilizing the spine to the pelvis, or the pelvis to the femur. Those most commonly involved are the sciatic, iliohypogastric, ilioinguinal, and lateral femoral cutaneous nerves. Entrapment of nerves that have no muscular innervation will not produce atrophy. Sensory dysfunction occurs either as hypoesthesia or hyperesthesia, depending on the severity of the neuropathy and its duration. Sciatic neuropathy may be accompanied by peripheral motor changes that closely resemble those produced by the radiculopathy of a herniated disc, but with it, the gluteal musculature is spared. Blockage of the suspected nerve markedly reduces pain. Even so, differentiating neuropathy and a disc herniation between L4-5 and L5-S1 is difficult. If blockage brings only transient relief, then neurolysis is probably indicated to relieve the neuropathy. Since neuropathy often causes and reinforces postural abnormality, its removal by neurolysis may relieve the postural stress as well, permitting recompensation of the stabilization system and relieving local as well as radiating pain.

The management of a low-back derangement is divided into two parts; the first is alleviation of the presenting episode. Then the conditions that permitted the derangement to occur should be helped. A program to maintain good health of the relevant myoligamentous structures is important. Although the patient should avoid sudden and violent low-back stress, too much pampering or imposed crippling will result in muscular weakness. A regime of regular bodily activity is important to promote the muscular synergy which is fundamental for normal back function.

index			
1	2	3	4
5	6	7	8
9	10		

index

A Abdomen, arteritis in, 68
  bloating of, 172
  hemorrhage from, 68
  pain in, obscure, 67-72
  perforation of, 68
Abreaction, 98
Abscess, subdiaphragmatic, 71
Acetazolamide, 90
Acid Cloak Creme®, 142
Acid, stomach, 75
Acidolate®, 137
Aci-Jel®, 185
Acne, 127-129
ACTH, 51
Addison's disease and hypotension, 10
Adenoids, enlarged, in snoring, 4, 5
Adenoma, thyroid, 24
Adenomyosis, 170
Adenopathy, preauricular, 83
Adolescence, 38, 127, 139
Adrenal gland, disorders of, and abdominal pain, 68
  hormones (see hormones)
  hyperfunction, 24, 68
  insufficiency, 24, 25, 26, 68
Adrenalin®, 122, 123
Aerophagia (see air-swallowing)
Age, role of, in snoring, 4
Agent (see class of agent or specific agent)
Agitation, 102
Air pollution, emphysema from, 45
Air-swallowing in infants, 36
Alcohol, and ulcer, 74
  as cause of snoring, 4
  excessive use of, 18, 24, 100
Allergy, 47-51
  and atopic dermatitis, 130
  and coughing, 55
  and foul breath, 6
  and postnasal drip, 58
  and toxic erythema, 147
  bacterial, 44
  differentiated from common cold, 56-57
  drug, 51
  gastrointestinal, 34
  nasal, 56
  penicillin, 51
  tests for, 48-51
Alpha-Keri®, 142
Amitriptyline, 107
Amphetamine, 11
Amyl nitrate, 91
Amyloidosis, 70
Analgesics, 61, 157, 174
  (see also specific drug)
Anemia, 18
  iron-deficiency, 24, 25, 26
  pernicious, 24, 25, 26, 67, 134
  sickle-cell, 24, 70
Aneurysm, dissecting, of aorta, 71
  of circle of Willis, 89
Anger, 100, 116
Angina, abdominal, 71
  Vincent's, organisms of, 7
Anorexia, 102, 103
Antacids, 73, 74

Antibiotics, 61, 83, 91
  (see also specific drug)
  candidiasis from, 184
  for acne, 128
  for atopic dermatitis, 132
  for endocarditis, 69
  for foot infections, 152
  for pharyngeal infections, 7
  for simple wounds, 121
  for sinusitis, 62
  overuse of, 31
  prophylactic use of, 32
Anticholinergics, 73, 74
  toxic reaction from, 69
Anticoagulants, hypoprothrombinemic, 69
  for venous occlusion, 90
Antidepressants, 105, 106, 174
  (see also specific drug)
Antifungal agents, 151, 152, 153
  (see also specific agent)
Antigens for allergy tests, 47-51
Antihistamines, 19, 57
  for snoring, 5
Antipruritics, 132
Antispasmodics, 73, 174, 195
Anxiety, 20, 95-98, 110, 115, 172, 174, 177
  abnormal, 96
  management of, 97, 98
  normal, 96
  physiological changes from, 95, 96
  recognition of, 96, 97
Aortic stenosis and hypotension, 10
Aphthae, oral (see canker sores)
Appetite, loss of, 21, 25
  (see also anorexia)
  variations in, in children, 30
Arches, fallen, 156
Argyrol®, 7
Arrhythmia, cardiac, 71
Arsenicals, 185 (see also specific drug)
  dermatitis from, 185
Arteriosclerosis, 177
  lack of, in low blood pressure, 9
Arteritis, necrotizing, in abdomen, 68
Arthritis, rheumatoid, 24
Aspirin, sensitivity to, 44
  toxic reaction from, 69
Asthma, 32, 43-46, 47, 49, 56
  and atopic dermatitis, 131
  atopic, 43-46
  bronchial, 48
  intrinsic, 44
  nonatopic, 43-46
Athlete's foot, 151-153
Atrophy, cavernous optic, 89
Atropine, 19, 84
Aureomycin®, 135
Avitaminosis, 24, 102 (see also vitamins)
Azotemia, 24

B Bacitracin, 86
Back, low, pain of, 193-196
Back pain, 102, 193-196
Bacteremia, 69
Baker's P&S Liquid®, 138

index

Barbiturates, 19
Basal metabolism rate in chronic hypertension, 9
Bed rest and hypotension, 11
Bed-wetting, 114-117
Behavior, antisocial, 173
Behcet's syndrome, 134
Benactyzine, 107
Biliary disease, 70
Biopsy, 164
   annular, 164
   coning, 164, 165
   for breast lesions, 168
   ring, 164
Blank, Irvin H., 141
Bleeding (see *hemorrhage*)
Blindness, night, 79
Blood, counts in hypotension, 9
   disorders (see specific disorder)
   loss of, from stomach and intestines, 24
      from uterus, 24
   pressure, low, 9-11 (see also *hypotension*)
   sugar, in hypotension, 9
Bowel, perforation of, 72
   ulceration of, 72
Bowlegs in children, 31
Boys (see *children*)
Bradycardia, 101
Brain, arteriosclerotic disease of, 20
   tumor of, 24
Breast, carcinoma of, 167, 168
   cystic disease of, 166
   fibroadenoma of, 168
   inflammation of (see *mastitis*)
   lumps in, 166-168
   swelling of, 172
Breath, foul, 6-8
Bromides, 129
Bromism, 24
Bronchiectasis, 24
   and foul breath, 7
   chronic, and coughing, 54, 55
Bronchitis, chronic, and foul breath, 7
Bronchodilators, 45, 46
   nebulized, 44
Brucellosis, 24
Budd-Chiari syndrome, 71
Bunion, 155
Burow's solution, 152
Bursitis over os calcis, 157

C Caffeine and ulcer, 74
Calcium for ear noises, 19
Caldwell, B. M., 180
Callus, 155, 156, 157
Calorie, expenditure, 28
   needs in children, 37
Cancer, 177 (see also *carcinoma*)
   lung, and coughing, 54
Candida albicans, 153
   infection with, 183, 184
Canker sores, 133-135
Carbasone®, 185
Carcinoma (see also *cancer*)
   bronchogenic, 24

Carcinoma, of breast, 167, 168
   of cecum, 24, 72
   of cervix, 163, 164
   of kidney, 24, 70
   of liver, 24
   of pancreas, 24, 72
   of right colon, 72
Carcinomatosis and hypotension, 10
Cardiac output, diminished, and hypotension, 10
Cardiovascular disorders (see specific disorder)
   and hypotension, 10
Carlson, A. J., 74
Cataracts, 79, 81, 87, 88, 90
Cecum, carcinoma of, 24
Cellulitis, 151
Cerumen, and coughing, 52
   and ear noises, 17
Cervix, benign erosion of, 163-165
   carcinoma of, 163, 164
   eversion of, 163
   inflammation of, 163, 164
      chronic, 164
      cystic, 164
   leukorrhea of, 163
Childbirth, weakness after, 25
Children, alleged growth problems in, 37-40
   neglectable disorders in, 30-32
   skin rash in, 143-147
   so-called colic in, 33-36
Chloramphenicol, 86
Chlordantoin cream, 185
Chlordiazepoxide hydrochloride, 98
Chlorisondamine, 192
Chlorothiazide, toxic reaction from, 69
Chlorpromazine, 98
Cholecystitis, 71
Cholestasis, extrahepatic, 69
Chronic brain syndrome, 20
Cleft tongue, 6, 8
Clostridium organisms, 121
Cocaine, diagnostic use of, 57
Cochlear mechanism, irritation of, 17
Colic, gallbladder, 71
   so-called, in infants, 33-36
Colon, carcinoma of, 24
   irritable, 13
   spastic, 15
Colpomicroscopy, 165
Colposcopy, 165
Common cold, differentiated from allergy, 56, 57
   and postnasal drip, 58
Complaints, about eyes, 79-91
   about mind and emotions, 95-117
   about respiratory system, 43-63
   about stomach, 67-75
   about the feet, 151-160
   about the skin, 127-147
   difficult-to-manage, 189-196
   "nuisance," 3-40
   peculiar to women, 163-185
Compulsions, 20
Congestion, hepatic, 70
Conjunctivitis, 80, 83, 84, 91

Constipation, 12-16, 102
   associated with hypotension, 11
Contactants, allergy to, 131
   (see also *allergy*)
Cornea, abrasion of, 85
   diseases of, 83
   inflammation of, 85, 86
   scarring of, 90
   ulcer of, 85
Corns, 151, 155, 157
Corsets, abdominal, for hypotension, 11
Corticosteroids, 128 (see also *steroids* and specific drug)
   for canker sores, 135
   for eye inflammation, 90
   for hypocalcemia, 70
   for psoriasis, 139
Cortisone, 25
   for atopic dermatitis, 132
Cough, chronic, 24, 45, 52-55, 56
Crying in infants, 34
Cuts, 121-124
Cyst, nabothian, 164
   subglottic, 53

D Dandruff, 136-139
Deafness, nerve, 17
Decongestants, nasal, 57
   ocular, 91
Delusions, 101
Dental problems, 177
Dentures, poorly fitting,
     and canker sores, 134
   and snoring, 4
Deoxypyridoxine, 139
Depression, 20, 21, 110, 172
   agitated, 101, 106
   and organic illness, 103
   diagnosis, 99-103
   examining for, 100
   in menopause, 181
   in the elderly, 106
   involutional, 101, 103
   manic-depressive disease, 103
   psychotic, 101, 102
   reactive, 101, 102
   treatment of, 104-107
Deprol®, 107
Dermatitis, atopic, 47, 130-132, 140
   chronic, 140
   circumscribed (see *lichen simplex*)
   contact, 130, 151
   from arsenicals, 185
   seborrheic, 130, 136, 137, 138, 139, 142
   "sheet," 140
Dermatosis, "diaper," 143, 144
Desensitization, histamine, 19
Developmental variations in children, 30
Dexamethasone, 128
Dextroamphetamine, 98
Diabetes mellitus, 11, 24, 25, 26, 32, 67, 72, 89, 177, 184
Diarrhea, 56, 68, 145
Dichlorphenamide, 90
Diet, 10
   and canker sores, 133
   and dandruff, 139

Diet, for premenstrual tension, 173
   rules for, 27-29
   trouble staying on, 27-29
Diethylstilbesterol, 181
Digitalis, toxic reaction from, 69
Diiodohydroxyquin, 185
Dilatation and curettage, 164
Disease (see specific disease or disorder)
Disorders (see specific disorder or disease)
Diuretics, 174 (see also specific drug)
Dizziness, 102
Domol®, 142
Drowsiness, 25
Drug, addiction to, 69
   eruptions, 134
Drugs (see class of drug or specific drug)
Drüsen, 88
Dry skin, 101, 140-142, 144, 146
Dryness of mouth, 103
Dysmenorrhea, 169-171
Dyspareunia, 183
Dysplasia in breast, 166

E Ear, infection of, 17, 18
Ear noise, 17-19
Eating as cause of snoring, 4
Eczema, 47, 56
   (see also *contact dermatitis*)
   contact, 47
   hand, 131, 151
   housewife's, 131
   infantile, 44, 131
   nummular, 131
Edema, 172
   vulval, 183
Elavil®, 107
Electrocauterization, 165
Embolism, mesenteric, 69
   pulmonary, 69, 71
   splenic, 69
Embolus and ischemia, 71
Emotional stress (see *stress*)
Emotions, and postnasal drip, 59
   complaints about, 95-117
   (see also *mind*)
   disturbances, 95-117, 177
   (see also specific emotion)
Emphysema, from air pollution, 45
   obstructive pulmonary, chronic 43-46
Encephalopathy, 192
Endocarditis, 24
   bacterial, 69
Endocervix, 164
   inflammation of, 163
Endocrine disturbances
   (see specific disturbance)
   and hypotension, 10
   as cause of snoring, 4
Endometriosis, 179
Endometrium and dysmenorrhea, 169-171
Enuresis (see *bed-wetting*)
Eosinophilia, 47, 48
   blood, in asthma, 43, 44, 45

Eosinophilia, in allergy, 57
  sputum, in asthma, 43, 45
Ephedrine, 11, 19
Epilepsy, 24
Epinephrine, 44, 46
  nebulized, 46
Epiphyses, closure of, 39
Epsom salts, 157
Erosion, acquired cervical, 163-165
  congenital cervical, 163-165
Erythema, periumbilical, 145, 146
  toxic, 146, 147
Erythema multiforme, 134
Erythrasma, 151
Erythrocytosis, symptomatic, 70
Estrogen, 171, 174, 176, 177, 180,
    181, 182, 184
  cream for vaginitis, 185
  for ozena and foul breath, 7
  therapy for tall girls, 39
Ether, 98
Ethmoiditis, 61
Ethoxzolamide, 90
Ethyl chloride, 195
Eustachian tube, obstruction of, 17
Eyes, complaints about, 79-91
  imbalance of muscle of, 80
  inflammation of, 83-86
  lens of, 87
  pain of, 84
  spots before, 89
  trauma of, 85
Eyesight, complaints about, 79-82
Excoriations, self-inflicted,
    in infants, 146, 147
Exercise, 10
  as cause of snoring, 4
  for fallen arches, 156
  for ozena and foul breath, 7
Exophthalmos, 25
Extropion, cervical, 163

F Face, pain in, 60
Fatigue, 10, 172, 174, 177
  organic causes of, 23-26
  psychogenic, 20-22
Fear, 109, 110 (see also *anxiety*)
Fecal impaction and foul breath, 6
Feet, complaints about, 151-160
Fever, 25, 145
  allergic, 47
  and hypotension, 11
Fibroadenoma, breast, 168
Fibroids, intramural, 170
Fixation, fecal, 16
Flat feet in children, 31
Fluid, retention of, 173
Fluorescein, 83, 85
Fluorohydrocortisone, 11 (see also
    steroids and *corticosteroids*)
Foods, solid, for infants, 35
Foot problems in women, 154-157
Foreign body, in bronchial tree, 55
  in ear canal, 52
  in eye, 80, 83, 85, 86
  in larynx, 53
Formula for infants, artificial, 35

Formula for infants, hypoallergic, 34
  ideal, 36
Fostex Cream®, 137
Foul breath, 6-8
Frenum, upper labial, 31

G Gallbladder, disease of, 13
Ganglion, cervical, 59
Gangrene and foul breath, 7
Gargle, throat, 53
Gastric dilatation, acute,
    and foul breath, 6
Gastroenterostomy, 75
Gentian violet, 152, 153, 185
Girls (see *children*)
Glaucoma, 80, 81, 82, 83, 84, 87,
    89, 90, 177
Glucose tolerance, impaired, 26
Glycerine, 142, 159
Goiter, 26
  surgery for, 25
Gonadotropin, chorionic, 170
Gordon, Dan M., 79
Graves' disease, 24
Griseofulvin, 153
Growth, problems of, in children, 37-40
Guanethidine, 11, 191, 192
Guilt, 108, 109
Gums, unhealthy, and foul breath, 6
Gynecologic disorders, 163-185
    (see also specific disorder)

H Halos around lights, 81, 84
Hay fever, 44, 47, 49
  and atopic dermatitis, 131
Head, injuries of, and ear noise, 18
Headache, 24, 25, 56, 60, 72, 102, 172
Heart, arrhythmia, 71
  congestive failure of, 71
  disease, 71
  murmur, 32
Heel, painful, 157
Hemangioma, capillary, 31
  in larynx, 53
  raised, 31
Hemigastrectomy, 75
Hemochromatosis, 69
Hemorrhage, and hypotension, 10
  from abdomen, 68
  from cervix, 163
  macular, 81
  retroperitoneal, 71
  vitreous, 81, 89
Hemorrhoid, sentinel, 15
Hepatitis, 24, 71
  viral, 70
Hepatomegaly, 70
Herpangina, 134
Herpes simplex, 86, 133, 135
Herpes zoster, 70
Histoplasmin, sensitivity to, 50
Hives, 56
Homatropine, 192
Hormones (see also specific hormone
    or drug)
  adrenocorticotrophic, 51

index

Hormones, anabolic, 5
  androgenic, 129
    unnecessary use of, 38
  sex, 127
Hydralazine, 189, 190, 192
Hydrochlorothiazide, 189, 190
  toxic reaction from, 69
Hydrocortisone, 135
  for low-back pain, 194
  for ozena and foul breath, 7
  for pruritus, 153
Hypercalcemia, 69, 70
Hypergammaglobulinemia, 71
Hyperinsulinism, diabetogenic, 24, 26
  functional, 24, 67, 69, 72
  organic, 24
Hyperkeratosis of palms and hands, 140
Hyperlipemia, 69
Hyperparathyroidism, 67, 68
  primary, 24
Hyperplasia, in breast, 166
  mucoepithelial, 163
Hypertension, 18, 68, 89, 177, 189-192
  benign, 189, 190
  diastolic, 189
  familial, 190
  malignant, 189, 191
  overdosage of drugs for, 11
  portal, 71
Hyperthyroidism, 24, 25, 68, 174
Hypertonic syndrome in infants, 36
Hyphemia, 85
Hypnosis, 174
Hypochondriasis, 21, 108-110
  breath odor, 8
Hypoglycemia, 25, 98
  functional, 173
  nocturnal, 24
  reactive, 25, 72
Hypometabolism in snoring, 4
Hypotension, 26
  chronic, 9-11
  orthostatic, 10, 11
Hypothyroidism, 24, 25, 26, 68
  and atopic dermatitis, 130
  in snoring, 5
Hypovolemia and hypotension, 10

I Ichthyosis, 140
Ileum, hemorrhagic infarct in, 72
Imipramine, 107
Impotency, sexual, 102
Infants (see *children*)
Infarction, myocardial, 71
  splenic, 70
Infection (see also specific infection)
  and foul breath, 6
  bacterial, 57, 83, 151
  following biopsy, 168
  fungal, 151-153
  lung, 103
  monilial, 153
  nasal, 7, 17
  of ear, 17, 18
  renal tract, 24
  sinus, 5, 7, 17, 56, 60-63

Infection, skin, 103
  throat, 17
  Trichophyton rubrum, 153
  upper respiratory, 60, 83
  viral, 31, 57, 83
Inflammation, of breast, 166, 174
  of eye, 83-86
  of toe, 158
  peribronchial, 45
Inhibitors, carbonic anhydrase, 82
  monoamine oxidase, 106, 107
Injuries, slight, 121-124
Insomnia, 21, 25, 172, 177
Instability, vasomotor, 176
Insufficiency, cardiac, acute, 192
  venous, and hypotension, 11
Insulin, 51, 98
Intracranial tumors and ear noise, 18
Invasion, perineural, 70
Iodides for ear noise, 19
Iodine, Lugol's, 164
  rinse, for foul breath, 6
Iodochlorhydroxyquin, 153
Iritis, 83, 84, 85
Ischemia, intermittent mesenteric, 71
Isocarboxazid, 106, 107
Isopropylarterenol, 46

J Jackson, Chevalier, 52
Jaundice, neonatal, 145
Jejunum, hemorrhagic infarct in, 72
Jordon, Sara, 15

K Kenalog in Orabase®, 135
Keratitis, 83, 85
Keratolytic agents, 128
Kidney, carcinoma of, 24
  disease of, 24, 69, 70, 71
  neoplasm in, 26
Knock-knees in children, 31

L Laceration (see *cuts*)
Lacrimal sac, anastomosis of, 80
Lacrimation, 84
  excessive, 80
Lactic acid, 185
Lactobacillus, 135, 184
Laughlin, H. R., 108
Laxatives, excessive use of, 12-16
Leg, cramps in, 25
Leukemia, 24, 25, 26, 134
Leukopenia, 48
Leukorrhea, cervical, 163
Lichen simplex chronicus, 136, 138-139
Liver, carcinoma of, 24
  disorder of, and foul breath, 6, 7
  enlargement of, 70
  noninfectious disease of, 24
  polycystic disease of, 71
Lowila Emollient®, 142
Lozenges, throat, 53
Lubath®, 142
Lubriderm®, 142

Lung, abscess of, and foul breath, 6, 7
  disease of (see specific disease)
  tumor of, 24
Lupus erythematosis, systemic, 71
Lymphadenitis, 152
  tuberculous mesenteric, 70
  tuberculous retroperitoneal, 70
Lymphadenopathy, cervical, 134
  hyperplastic, 72
Lymphangitis, 152
Lymphoma, 24

M Macro-milia (see *milia*)
Macular disease, 87, 88, 90
Malabsorption, 24
  primary, 25
Malignancy (see also specific type of malignancy)
  cervical, 163, 164, 182
  ovarian, 182
Malnutrition, 24, 25
  and hypotension, 10
Marplan®, 107
Mass, breast (see *breast*)
Mastectomy, 168
Mastitis, chronic, 166
  chronic cystic, 174
Mecamylamine, 191, 192
Mediterranean fever, recurring, 69
Medroxyprogesterone, 171
Mellobath®, 142
Membrane, Bruch's, 88
Memory, changes in, 72
Menarche, premature, 39
Ménière's disease, 17
Menopause, hormonal management of, 180-182
  practical management of, 175-179
Menstruation, and allergy, 56
  disturbances in, 174
  painful, 169-171
Mental illness, 113 (see also *emotions* and specific symptom)
Meprobamate, 107
Metabolism, disorders of, 69 (see also specific disorder)
Metatarsus, 154, 155
Methamphetamine hydrochloride, 174
Methylene Blue, diagnostic use of, 59
Methyltestosterone, 181
Metronidazole, 184, 185
Meyer, Robert, 165
Middle ear, 17
Migraine, abdominal, 72
Milia, 145, 146
Mind, complaints about, 95-117 (see also *emotions*)
Miotic agents, 82, 90
Mirror, head, examination with, 61, 62
Monoamine oxidase inhibitors, 106, 107
Mononucleosis, infectious, 70
Mouth-breathing, 59
  and foul breath, 6
Mucosa, nasal, drying of, 59
Multiple myeloma, 24
Multiple sclerosis, 24
  and hypotension, 11

Muscle, relaxants for, 195
  tonus, decreased, 101
Myasthenia gravis, 24, 25
Mydriatics, 84
Myeloma, 70
  multiple, 24
Myocardial, infarction, and hypotension, 10
  insufficiency, and hypotension, 10
Myometrium and dysmenorrhea, 169-171
Myopathy, related to granulomatous, connective-tissue, and neoplastic disorders, 24
Myopia, 90

N Nalorphine, 69
Narcolepsy, 24, 25, 26
Nardil®, 107
Nausea, 84, 102, 172, 177
Neomycin, 86
Nerve, entrapment of, 195
  trigeminal, 59
Neurodermatitis (see *atopic dermatitis*)
Neuropathy, diffuse autonomic, 11
  peripheral, 11
Neurosis, 16, 20, 72, 95, 110, 174, 178
Neutropenia, cyclic, 134
Nialamide, 106, 107
Niamid®, 107
Nitrous oxide, 98
Nivea Creme®, 142
Nodules, hypertrophic lymphoid, 52
Noises, ear, 17-19
  offending, in snoring, 3
Norepinephrine, 106
  from pheochromocytoma, 68
Norethynodril, 171
Normality of children, 37
Nose, blockage of, and foul breath, 6
  deformities, in snoring, 4, 5
  discharge from, 60
  infection of, 7, 17
  mucosal drying of, 59
  obstruction of, 4, 60
  polyps of, 5, 47, 56, 61, 63
  stuffiness of, 47
Nose drops, 5, 53
Nutrition, improved, for ozena and foul breath, 7
Nystatin, 185

O Obesity, 27-29, 174
  health hazards of, 28
Obsessive-compulsive disorder, 95
Obstipation, 101
Obstruction, intestinal, 70
  nasal (see *nose*)
  ventilatory, 43
Occlusion, vascular, mesenteric, 71
Odor, breath, 6-8
Oil, use of, for skin dryness, 141, 142
Olfactory sense, acuteness of, 8
Omphalitis, 145
Osteoporosis, 181
Otosclerosis, 17
Ovary, insufficiency of, 24
Overweight, 27, 176 (see also *obesity*)

204 index

Oxytetracycline, 86
Ozena in foul breath, 7

P Pain, costovertebral, 68
    joint, 24
    low-back, 193-196
    obscure abdominal, 67-72
    ocular, 84
    upper left quadrant, 69
Palate, high, enlarged, in snoring, 4
Pancreas, carcinoma of, 24
    inflammation of, 68, 70, 71
    islet-cell tumor of, 26
    ulcerogenic tumor of, 68
Papilledema, 80
Paralysis, hyperkalemic, 24
    hypokalemic, 24
    normokalemic, 24
    periodic, 24
Paranoid tendencies, 101
Parkinsonism, 24
Pemphigus, 134
Penicillin, 51, 83
Penicilloyl polylysine, 51
Pentolinium, 192
Percentile grid, use of, 39, 40
Pericarditis, constrictive,
    and hypotension, 10
Peritonitis and foul breath, 6
Petrolatum, 142, 159
Pharynx, infection in, 7
    inflammation of, and foul breath, 6
Phenelzine, 106, 107
Phenobarbital, 190
Phenol mixed with salt for psoriasis, 139
Phenylbutazone, toxic reactions from, 69
Pheochromocytoma, 24, 68
Phobia, 20 (see also *fear* and *anxiety*)
Photophobia, 80, 83, 84
Pigmentation, cutaneous, 26
Pituitary, insufficiency of, 26
Placebo, 173
Pleuritis, diaphragmatic, 69
Pneumonia, 102
Poisoning, arsenic, 69
    lead, 69
Polyarteritis, 71, 72
Polyarthritis, 24
Polycythemia, 68
    vera, 70, 71
Polyps, nasal, 5, 44, 47, 56, 61, 63
    pedunculated laryngeal, 53
    sinus, 44
Porphyria, 69
Postnasal drip, 58, 59
    in foul breath, 7
    in snoring, 5
Potassium permanganate, 152
Pragmatar®, 137
Prednisolone, 135
Prednisone, 135
Pregnancy, and aortic aneurysm, 71
    and hypotension, 11
Premenstrual tension, 172-174
Pressor agents, 10

Procaine, 122, 160, 195
Progesterone, 170, 171, 174
Propionate compound and jelly, 185
Prostatism, unrecognized, 24
Protein-bound iodine in
    chronic hypotension, 9
Pruritus, vulval, 183
Pruritus senilis, 140
Pseudopregnancy, 170, 171
Psoriasis, 130, 136, 137, 138, 139, 151
Psychic factors (see *emotions*)
Psychophysiological disorders, 72
Psychosis, 16, 20, 174
Psychotherapy, 110
    for atopic dermatitis, 132
    for premenstrual tension, 173
Pustules, 146, 147
Pylorus, operation on, 75
Pyoderma, 144
Pyridoxine, deficiency of, 139

Q Quinine, 18

R Rash, diaper, 143, 144, 146
    maculopapular, 144, 145, 146
Rectocele, 15
Referral, psychiatric, 8, 53, 110, 111-113, 132, 173
Reflex, coughing, 52
    gastrocolic, 13, 14
Reflexes, hyperactive, in infants, 36
Refraction, error of, 80
Resection, wedge, for ingrown toenail, 158
Reserpine, 190, 192
    toxic reaction from, 69
Respiratory infection and emphysema, 45
Respiratory system, complaints about, 43-63
Respiratory tract, sensitivity of, 52
    upper, and foul breath, 6
Rest, proper, for ozena and foul breath, 7
Retina, detachment of, 81, 88
    occlusion of vessel, 81
Retinitis pigmentosa, 79
Retinoblastoma, 80
Rheumatic fever, 24, 32
Rheumatoid arthritis, 24
Rhinitis, allergic, 48
    as cause of snoring, 5
    atrophic, and foul breath, 7
    in snoring, 4, 5
    chronic, and coughing, 52
Rynearson, Edward H., 28

S Salicylates, 18, 195
Salicylic acid, for athlete's foot, 153
    for corns and calluses, 157
Salivation, decreased, 102
    impairment of, 11
Salt, increased intake,
    for hypotension, 11
    iodized, 129
    rinse for foul breath, 6, 7
    solution for sinusitis, 62

Sarcoidosis, 24
Schedules, feeding, for infants, 35
Schizophrenia, ambulatory,
   and abdominal pain, 72
  pseudoallergic, 72
Secretion, nasal, 58, 59
  postnasal, 58, 59
Sedatives, 73, 74 (see also specific drug)
  excessive use of, 100
  for atopic dermatitis, 132
Selsun®, 137
Sensitivity, drug, 50
Serotonin, 106
Serum sickness, 51
Sex, attitude towards, 178
  disturbances of, 172
Shearman, A. M., 181
Shelton, E. K., 181
Shoes, improperly fitting, 154-157
Sickle-cell Hemoglobin C disease, 70
Silicone, 144
Silver nitrate, 53, 165
Silver picrate, 185
Simmond's disease, 10
Sinuses, anatomy of, 60
  infection of, 5, 7, 17, 56, 60-63
    chronic, and coughing, 52
    frontal, 60, 61
    maxillary, 61
    sphenoidal, 61
Sjögren syndrome, 67
Skin, complaints about, 127-147
  dryness of, 140-142
    in infants, 144, 146
  infection (see specific infection)
  pigmentation of, 68
  tingling of, 177
Skin rash, 130-132
  "diaper," 143, 144, 146
  in infants, 143-147
  maculopapular, 144, 145, 146
  neonatal, 143-147
Skin testing, 44
  for allergy, 131
Sleep, disturbances of, 72 (see also *insomnia*)
Smallpox inoculation for canker sores, 135
Smear, Papanicolaou, 163, 164, 165, 184
  wet, for vaginitis, 184
Smoking, as cause of snoring, 4
  excessive, 45 (see also *tobacco*)
Snoring, 3-5
Sodium amytal, 98
Sodium bicarbonate for douches, 185
Sodium chloride, 180 (see also *salt*)
Soft palate, vibration of, in snoring, 3
Soporific drugs, 105
Spinal anesthesia and hypotension, 10
Spine, lumbar, derangement of, 193
Sprays, medicinal, overuse of, 59
Spur, calcaneal, 157
Staphylococci, 50, 147
Staphylococcus aureus, 185
Steroid, 91 (see also *corticosteroid* and specific drug)
  adrenocortical, 44, 45, 46, 68, 70
    toxic reaction from, 69

Steroid, for atopic dermatitis, 132
  for dysmenorrhea, 170, 171
  for eye inflammation, 86
  for iritis, 84
  for lichen simplex, 139
  sex, 180
Stockings, elastic, for hypotension, 11
Stomach, acid in, 75
  complaints about, 67-75
  resection of, 75
  rest of, for ulcer, 73-75
Strabismus, nonparalytic, 80
Streptococci, 50, 147
Stress, emotional, and allergy, 47
  and asthma, 46
  and atopic dermatitis, 130
  and canker sores, 133
  and ear noise, 19
Strokes, little, 24, 25, 72
Suicide, 21, 104, 105, 107, 173
Sulfa drugs for pharyngeal infection, 7
Surgery, for ingrown toenail, 158-160
  office, for simple lacerations, 121-124
Sweats, night, 24
Sympathetic nervous system and hypotension, 11
Sympathomimetic drugs, 192
Sympathoplegic drugs, 11
Syndrome (see specific syndrome)
Syphilis, 71
  secondary, 151
Syringomyelia and hypotension, 11

T Tachycardia, 25
Taste, bad, 72
Tear ducts, probing of, 80
Teeth, decayed, and foul breath, 6, 7
  natural and artificial, and foul breath, 6
  permanent, in children, 31
Tension, 110 (see also *emotions*)
  in expectant mothers, 33
  premenstrual, 172-174
Test, intradermal, for allergy, 49
  patch, for allergy, 48
  Schiller, 164
  scratch, for allergy, 48
Tetanus antitoxin, 121, 124
  human, antitoxin, 122
  toxoid, 122
Tetracycline, 86, 128
Tetrahydrozoline, 91
Theophylline, 46
Throat, infection of, 17
Thrombosis, mesenteric, 70, 71
  of hepatic veins, 71
  of portal vein, 71
Thyroid extract, 5
Thyroiditis, 67
Tincture of green soap, 137
Tinea capitis, 153
Tinea cruris, 153
Tinnitus, 17-19
Tissue, heteroplastic endocervical, 163
Tobacco, and postnasal drip, 58
  and ulcer, 74
  excessive use of, 18, 54

Toe, inflammation of, 158
Toenail, ingrown, 158-160
Tofranil®, 107
Tongue, burning of, 72
  cleft, and foul breath, 6
Tongue-tie, 31
Tonics, appetite-stimulating, 30
  for depression, 106
  unnecessary use of, 38
Tonsils, enlarged, in snoring, 4, 5
  infected, and foul breath, 7
  unnecessary removal of, 31
Tracheitis and coughing, 53
Tranquilizers, 19, 105, 106, 174
Transillumination of sinuses, 62
Trauma, eye, 85
Trench mouth, 134
Triamcinolone, 128, 135
Trichloroacetic acid, 135
Trichomoniasis, 183, 184
  (see also *vaginitis*)
Trichophyton rubrum, 152
Tuberculin, sensitivity to, 50
Tuberculosis, 24, 26, 54, 70, 177
Tubules, Skene's, 184
Tumor, abdominal, 71
  extramedullary, 70
  retroperitoneal, 24

U Ulcer, anal, chronic, 15
  corneal, 80, 102
  duodenal, 68, 177
  gastric, 177
  jejunal, 68
  peptic, 68, 70, 71, 72, 73-75
  skin, 102
  stomach, 68
  toe, 158
Umbilical hernia, 31
Underweight in patients
  with hypotension, 10
Upper respiratory tract, bleeding in, 7
  infection of (see *infection*)
Urea, 82
Urination, burning during, 183
  difficult, 11
  frequent, 177
Urticaria, 47, 51
Uveitis, 81, 83, 84
Uvula, amputation of, 53
  elongated and edematous,
    in coughing, 53
  in snoring, 4, 5
  vibration of, in snoring, 3

V Vaginitis, atrophic, 183
  bacterial, 184, 185
  Candida (monilial), 183
  infectious, 183-185
  Trichomonas vaginalis, 183
Vagotomy, 75
Varicosities, venous, and hypotension, 11
Vasodilators, 79
Vermilion halo, 163
Vertebrae, osteoporotic, collapse of, 68
Vincent's angina, organisms of, 7
Viral infections, 31, 32
Vision, blurring of, 80, 91
  deficiency of field, 80, 81
  failing, in the elderly, 87-91
  loss of, 81, 88
  tunnel, 88
Vital capacity in asthma, 44
Vitamin A, deficiency of, 79
  for ozena and foul breath, 7
  intoxication from, 24
Vitamin B, 19
Vitamin B_{12} for ozena
  and foul breath, 7
Vitamin D, for ozena
  and foul breath, 7
  intoxication from, 24
Vitamins, appetite-stimulating, 30
  deficiency of, 24, 102
  for acne, 129
  for depression, 106
  for premenstrual tension, 174
  multiple, 5
Vomiting, 84
  cyclic, 56

W Wasting disease and hypotension, 10
Weight, gain in, 172
  loss of, 25, 27-29, 102, 103
"Winter itch," 140
Women, complaints peculiar to, 163-185

X X-ray, for abdominal pain, 67
  of sinuses, 62
  therapy for acne, 129
  therapy for canker sores, 135
Xylocaine Viscous Syrup®, 135

Z Zephiran®, 123
Zollinger-Ellison syndrome, 68